Geopathic Stress
&
Subtle Energy

Copyright © 2006   Jane Thurnell-Read
Drawings by Irvin Klein, California, USA

ISBN: 0 9542439 4 3

Published by:

Life-Work Potential
Sea View House
Long Rock
Penzance
Cornwall
TR20 8JF
England

Tel: + 44 (0)1736 719030
Fax: + 44 (0)1736 719040
www.lifeworkpotential.com

Geopathic Stress
&
Subtle Energy

Jane Thurnell-Read

Other books by the author:

Health Kinesiology: The Muscle Testing System That Talks To The Body
ISBN 0 9542439 0 0, Life-Work Potential, 2002

The Guide To Geopathic Stress
ISBN 1 84333 529 8, Vega, 2002 (no longer in print)

Verbal Questioning Skills For Kinesiologists
ISBN 0 9542439 19, Life-Work Potential, 2004

Energy Mismatch
ISBN: 0 9542439 35, Life-Work Potential, 2004

Allergy A To Z
ISBN: 0 9542439 2 7, Life-Work Potential, 2005

Visit

www.healthandgoodness.com
for information, tips and inspiration
for a happier, healthier life

also

www.mytherapypractice.com
for information for practitioners

(Both web sites have associated free monthly online
newsletters – don't forget to sign up)

INTRODUCTION

My first book on geopathic stress entitled *Geopathic Stress: How Earth Energies Affect Our Lives* was published in 1994 and was well received. It had been out of print for several years when I decided to update it in 2005. Although I no longer practised as a geopathic stress consultant, I knew that many people were keen to see the book back in print.

At first I thought this would be a quick task but, as I came to read what I had previously written and to research what practitioners are doing currently, the book began to change. By early 2006 I realised that, although much of the material was still relevant, I was writing a new book – a book on geopathic stress and subtle energy – and that it needed a different title to reflect the difference in emphasis. Once I had realised all this the title was obvious – *Geopathic Stress & Subtle Energy*.

My original interest in geopathic stress came about as a result of inconsistencies I was finding in my own natural health care practice. I helped many clients with a whole range of symptoms and illnesses, both physical and psychological, but there was a group of clients who did not respond to treatment. I did not expect to be successful with everyone, but I had developed an instinct for knowing the people I would be able to help. It would have been easy to dismiss these people as hypochondriacs, who did not want to get better, but it was very clear to me that many of them did not fall into this category. I began to wonder if geopathic stress was the missing factor. When I started correcting geopathic stress problems, I found that some of these clients with seemingly intractable problems started to get better.

I no longer work as a practitioner, but concentrate on research and writing for articles, books, and my web sites for the public and for students and practitioners. I also spend time researching and developing test kits for therapists. A lot of what I write is very practical and based on giving people simple, easy ways they can help themselves, or information on how complementary therapies can help them. But a continuing background interest has been in something more nebulous - the nature of 'subtle energy'. Writing this book has allowed me to explore this concept of subtle energy in more depth than is usual in my writing.

Both terms 'geopathic stress' and 'subtle energy' are difficult to pin down. Are geopathic energies part of the electromagnetic spectrum? Or are they something altogether more 'subtle'? What is the nature of subtle energy? Is quantum mechanics approaching the idea of subtle energy by another name? It would be foolish to claim that I have the answers to these important questions, but in writing this book I have tried to tackle these questions with an open, inquisitive and intelligent mind.

This book does not claim to be totally comprehensive. There are competent and successful practitioners who are not included. There are many devices on the market to counteract geopathic stress and electromagnetic pollution and not all of them are discussed here.

CHAPTER 1

An Overview

Origins Of The Term

Geopathic comes from two Greek words: *geo* means 'of the earth', and *pathos* means 'suffering' or 'disease'. The word 'geopathic' literally means suffering or disease of the earth. Geopathic stress (GS) is the general term for energies emanating from the earth that cause discomfort and ill health in human beings. Because of their detrimental effect, they are often known as negative earth energies.

Some people use the term geopathic stress only to describe ley lines (man-made energy lines, see page 47), or only to describe energy disturbances caused by underground water (see page 39). Yet others use the term in a way that includes both energy disturbances from the earth and man-made electromagnetic pollution such as power lines, radio waves, and so on (see appendix 1). People who restrict the meaning to either ley lines or underground water will miss many energies that have a destructive effect on people's health. On the other hand widening the concept of geopathic stress to include electromagnetic pollution can be misleading and confusing.

The Beginnings

Initial interest in the idea of geopathic stress was stimulated by the work of Winzer and Melzer in Germany in the 1920's. In

Stuttgart they found geological faults present in the areas of the city with the highest incidence of cancer. Gustav Freiherr von Pohl took this work further and studied two places: Vilsbiburg and Grafenau. Vilsbiburg had a very high incidence of cancer and Grafenau a very low incidence. In Vilsbiburg von Pohl accurately predicted the incidence of cancer by dowsing for 'water veins' using a 1:1,000 scale map of the town. This survey was greeted with some scepticism because Vilsbiburg was a small town (8,300 inhabitants) with a high cancer rate. Von Pohl then turned his attention to Grafenau, which was the town with the lowest incidence of cancer in the area. Once again von Pohl showed a link between cancer cases and geopathic zones. (Christopher Bird, *The Divining Hand*).

The Effects

There are many different types of geopathic energies with some people being more susceptible than others. Sleeping, living or working constantly in a geopathically stressed area can lead to emotional and physical problems and difficulties, which exact a heavy toll on both the sufferers and their families. Cancers, miscarriages, chronic ill health and personality changes have all been linked to geopathic stress.

Unfortunately, because most people do not know about geopathic stress, they do not realise what is happening. They do not know that it is possible to make changes that can neutralise the effect of these negative earth energies and allow people to avoid serious ill-health, or re-gain previous good health and well-being.

If exposure to geopathic energies is short-lived, the effects are usually insignificant, although some people will show symptoms of tiredness, inattention and headaches when sitting in a particular geopathically stressed area for even one or two hours. Inattentiveness in long meetings is not necessarily a sign of boredom. An engineer once challenged me to assess a lecture theatre for geopathic energies and then predict who would experience headaches or lethargy during an afternoon lecture by him. During his lecture he asked people to raise their hand if they had a headache or felt unwell in some way. Many of the people who did were sitting in the seats I had designated. My engineering friend was very impressed by the result.

Any effect from short-term exposure such as this is likely to be transitory. The body quickly recovers and returns to its normal state. Problems only occur when people spend a long time in places where the earth's energy is disturbed, perhaps when an individual's house or work place (or sometimes even both) is in an area of high geopathic stress.

Shortage Of Building Land

As building land becomes increasingly scarce, there is less and less choice about where houses are built. Even if builders and architects had an understanding of GS there would be fewer and fewer options about where to put houses and other buildings. As it is, the location of buildings is determined on purely commercial grounds, taking into account land prices, proximity to transport, planning rules and so on. The day when building sites are routinely assessed for geopathic stress is a long way off.

People may live in the same building for many years, and their exposure to a particular form of negative energy can last a long time. Rolf Gordon, the founder of the Dulwich Health Society (13), has remarked that gypsies very rarely get cancer. Gordon believes this is because they move from place to place, so that their exposure to a 'bad' place would only be for a couple of weeks at most. He also notes that when choosing a site gypsies take into account the feel of a place. There is no conclusive proof that the reason there is so little cancer among gypsies is because their exposure to geopathic influences is kept to a minimum, but it is an interesting theory. Some writers have suggested that in more 'primitive' times, humans had some understanding of these matters and so would build appropriately, taking into account the feel of the land.

The Evidence

I have used case studies for illustration throughout the book. Unfortunately these do not convince the scientific mind. When I talk to some of my scientific friends, they tell me I am citing anecdotal evidence. While accepting that this is true, it does not mean that the anecdotes are wrong or unworthy of consideration. As we amass more of these, the evidence becomes increasingly persuasive. Sceptics seem to be particularly impressed by the fact that animals are also affected by geopathic energies (see page 15 and 22), and it is hoped there will be more well documented case studies in this area.

Predictive studies also give the sceptic food for thought. (See pages 18, 19 and 77 for examples of these.) Of course, illness can occur even when geopathic stress is not present, so there is not a total correlation between geopathic stress and illness. Most critics who dismiss the concept of geopathic stress out of hand are taken aback when they see how it can be used predictively. This is much more convincing than producing evidence that people pay a practitioner money to fix their houses and then get better. The sceptic mutters: 'Placebo effect' or: 'They got better because they paid you'. When a practitioner can accurately predict problems, the sceptic may still not accept the idea of geopathic stress, but they usually accept that the practitioner has produced an accurate prediction in a way that they cannot explain.

A study using live blood analysis conducted at Wageningen University in the Netherlands in 2005 offers an alternative type of evidence. A blood sample was taken from a woman before she had a Geomack unit installed (see page 111). This sample showed that the red blood cells were in long chains – the Rouleau effect.

This severely reduces the surface area of the red blood cells, and so makes these vital cells much less efficient. Another blood sample was taken twelve weeks later. In the mean time the woman had made no other changes - her house, her diet, her medication, etc. were the same. This blood sample showed very little evidence of the Rouleau effect, meaning that the red blood cells were now able to perform more efficiently.

Ann and Roy Procter (30), who correct geopathic problems without visiting the site, carried out an interesting study. The results were presented at the International Conference in Manchester organised by the British Society of Dowsers (07) in August 2003. The paper was subsequently published in two parts in *Dowsing Today* (Vol 40 nos. 282 & 283). It can also be found on the Procters' web site (30). They enlisted the help of Dr Vicky Wass, who was a tutor in statistics in the Business School at Cardiff University, Wales. She helped design the questionnaires and analysed the results.

The research was carried out with the help of 105 households that had requested the Procters' help (in serial order as they came in, with no exceptions) for problems that they believed were associated with geopathic stress and/or discarnate presences (see page 51). Each household was asked to complete four identical questionnaires. The questionnaire asked about 26 personal and house-related symptoms. The first questionnaire was completed before any work was undertaken.

The respondents were then divided into two groups for the second questionnaire. One group received the questionnaire after the work had been done, and the other group, effectively a control group, before the work was done. No one knew which group they were in, and neither did Dr Wass, who was carrying out the statistical analysis. The third questionnaire was sent after the work had been completed and the fourth about a month later. Of the initial 150 households 105 households completed all four surveys. At the end of the survey 85 of the 105 respondents "showed, by their filling of the questionnaires, that they experienced some improvement in health".

What makes this study even more interesting is the responses to the second questionnaire. 16 respondents in the control group said they had benefited, even before anything had been done. 48 of the other group reported a benefit – they completed the questionnaire after the work had been done. The 16 members of the control group who benefited presumably would have improved anyway, or they experienced a placebo effect. This suggests that, of the 48 in the second group who benefited, 16 of them would have reported a benefit even if nothing had been done. This indicated that 32 of them had received some real, immediate benefit. These numbers increased with time, as the effect of the work brought about healing for more people. This is an ingenious study and deserves to be much more widely known.

Although understanding of geopathic stress is still incomplete, it is possible to make dramatic differences to some people's lives by taking these energies into account. We cannot stand back and wait for full understanding and proof, because many people's lives and health are being damaged daily by these phenomena.

Positive Earth Energies

It is important to understand that not all earth energies are negative. In fact a few practitioners would say that none are unless humans intervene. The majority of experts in this field do believe that some earth energies are problematic in their own right, but also recognise that some earth energies can be beneficial.

I took a friend to an area of high geopathic stress and he said that he really liked it because it made him feel very calm and peaceful. He is a man who finds it difficult to relax and is always on the go with new ideas and projects. He experienced the lowering effect as calming. This benefit would, however, only be short-term. With continuous exposure he too would almost certainly experience ill health and lack of energy.

However, this does suggest a way in which earth energies can be used in the future. It may be possible to manipulate the energies of individual rooms so that we can have rooms which offer a calming and relaxing experience for sleeping and resting, and a more stimulating energy for spaces in which work takes place. This would take into account the feng shui concepts of yin and yang (see appendix 3). A bedroom would require more yin characteristics, whereas an office space would probably need to be more yang. Each room would have its individual 'energy thermostat' so that the energy in the room could be adjusted in the same way that the temperature and the lighting can be today. Whether we can (or even should) harness earth energies in this way remains to be seen.

Even now some therapists carry out healing procedures on their clients at particular spots that they believe will enhance the healing potential of their work. Some geopathic consultants seek to enhance positive earth energies as well as removing and transforming negative ones.

Some years ago I put together seven earth energy essences. The essences (Balance, Comfort, Energy & Realism, Inner Wisdom, Need, Pain and Space) are a combination of place, time of day, season, sea-state, weather and prevailing mood. They have been 'collected' from various places in west Cornwall (UK) where I live. These essences use the earth's energy in a positive way to enhance health and life. Some practitioners use them as part of a treatment, but they can also be 'taken'. The usual way to do this is to place one drop of the appropriate essence on the webbing between the thumb and the first finger of the left hand. (Appendix 4 gives a full repertory of these essences.)

Limited Knowledge

Clearly, our knowledge in this field is limited, but this does not mean that these energies do not exist. The existence of geopathic energy can be inferred from its effect on humans, animals and plants. Much of our knowledge in physics and biology is, at least initially, inferred: the existence of phenomena is extrapolated from what can be seen and measured in the every day world. Models are produced which suggest a certain thing must happen or be there because of the resulting activity, even though the process or phenomenon cannot itself be mapped.

Geopathic energy is an insidious phenomenon: we cannot see it or adequately explain it in current scientific terms. Geopathic energies pass through floors, through windows and through closed doors - they do not recognise boundaries, walls or fences. Geopathic energies are not fixed and stable - they may change according to the season or time of day. They may also change because of building work, even if it is being carried out in a house some way off. Geopathic energies can be distorted and transferred to buildings other than where the work is taking place.

Perhaps one day it will become commonplace to have a geopathic survey done on a new house, or building site. If necessary, remedial action would then have to be taken by the owner or builder in order to ensure a sale. Similarly, it will hopefully become unthinkable to build a hospital on a site that has not been checked, or to make changes to the fabric of a school without looking at the energy implications.

CHAPTER 2

EFFECTS OF GEOPATHIC STRESS

There are many different ways in which geopathic stress can affect people, regardless of the source of the energy disturbance, but these are generally insidious - we do not suddenly drop dead or become ill after standing, sitting or sleeping on a particular spot. Nevertheless there are certain health problems that suggest that GS might be involved.

Disturbed Sleep Patterns & Tiredness

People who live in houses above areas of geopathic stress often have disturbed sleep patterns. They may not be able to get to sleep. They may wake frequently or suffer from strange dreams, so they wake feeling tired and irritable. As Michael and Maureen Rawles say on their web site (31):

> One of the 'Telltale Signs' of Geopathic Stress, is associated with 'sleeping long' and 'waking tired '.

This can lead to ill health, a lack of tolerance for others and general feelings of depression. In this situation arguments with loved ones ensue and life can become more and more difficult.

Babies and children in such houses may not sleep, so causing problems both for themselves and for their parents. They will often attempt to avoid sleeping in a geopathic area, and may be found in the morning scrunched up on one side or at one end of their bed. Unfortunately as we become older we become less aware of the problem and generally do not instinctively move away from it.

Of course, the sceptic will say that a lot of people feel tired and irritable a lot of the time, but susceptible individuals will report that they sleep better and are less tired once the geopathic energies are corrected.

Chronic Ill Health

Living or working over a geopathically stressed zone can lead a person to suffer from a whole range of different problems. Sadly, these people are often regarded as neurotics or hypochondriacs by the medical profession, their family and their friends. This adds to their overall stress levels, as they feel that no one really understands. Their symptoms become worse and worse and their health is more and more compromised. Alfred Riggs (32) told me he had worked with 3700 chronic fatigue cases in 22 countries, and his advice had led to a major improvement in the quality of life for most of these people.

Cancer & Multiple Sclerosis

Many serious complaints have been linked to geopathic stress, in particular cancer and multiple sclerosis. This is particularly true if the negative energy is found in the bedroom. It may well be that the disease would have developed eventually anyway, but the ongoing exposure to geopathic stress compounds the problems. Removing the GS will probably not cure the cancer, but it will allow the treatment of medical or alternative therapy or both, to be more effective. Rolf Gordon, the developer of the RadiTech (see page 114) told me about an interesting case of a small child with cancer who could not tolerate the full dose of chemotherapy. After a RadiTech was installed he was able to tolerate the full dose and made a complete recovery.

Miscarriages, Birth Defects & Infertility

When I checked the office described on page 18, I asked if there had been many miscarriages, as there were a lot of young female staff. The manager thought for a minute and then told me that there had not been many miscarriages, but nor had many babies been born to employees. She had not appreciated this before, but now was surprised that it was the case. We both wondered if some of these women had miscarried at an early stage, and had not told anyone at work. This was never taken any further, but it was remarkable how few women had become pregnant in that office.

Alfred Riggs (32) believes that many cases of sudden infant death syndrome are attributable to the mother sleeping in a problem area while the embryo is developing. He also cites cases where mothers gave birth to healthy babies and then had several miscarriages:

> I was able to correctly state in these circumstances that the healthy child was not conceived within the confines of that sleeping site, it further transpired that in all cases that they had slept in another bedroom I had previously checked without detecting any noxious radiation.

Allergies

When I worked as a practitioner, I had clients who appeared to be sensitive to many foods, chemicals, inhalants and contact substances. Some of these people were very sensitive to geopathic and man-made electromagnetic phenomena. The apparent 'allergies' were often low tolerance levels for these substances. When the sensitivity to these negative energies was reduced, their tolerance for a wide range of substances frequently increased dramatically. This was particularly likely in people who were suffering from chronic fatigue syndrome.

Failure To Respond To Treatment

My initial interest in this topic came about because I had clients who were not getting well, even though I felt they should, and this is agreed by practitioners in this field to be a good indicator of GS problems. Dr Robert Jacobs writing in the online magazine of the Wholistic Research Company (39) says:

> In my own practice I find that the main effect of Geopathic Stress is that it stops patients getting completely better. It appears to block the action of virtually any type of therapy. When patients tell me that they have already seen two homoeopaths, an acupuncturist, and three Harley Street consultants, none of whom could get them better I find that they are usually suffering from Geopathic stress.

Richard Gerber in *Vibrational Medicine* recounts tests using a Vega machine and a rotation tester, which showed changes in the blood of those exposed to geopathic stress. It had been found that these individuals had a counter clockwise rotational polarity in their blood. On moving away from these detrimental energies, the blood eventually developed the normal clockwise polarity again. While their blood exhibited this abnormal polarity, these people also seemed resistant to treatment for any chronic illness. He goes on to say that it has been shown that many cancer sufferers exhibit this counter clockwise polarity when tested using a Vega machine.

Psychological Problems

As well as physical problems, geopathic stress can cause psychological problems. At its simplest people whose sleep is disturbed by GS are likely to be less happy and less patient with others.

Mike and Maureen Rawles (31) have found that correcting negative earth energies can make a huge difference to people's psychological state, and so to their relationships. They gave me this example:

> A family moved into a different house, which made certain members reclusive, irrationally aggressive, and depressed. Investigations showed that the prior owners had never liked the house (in the three years they stayed), and that those in the house before them came close to divorce, before moving. Complex negative earth energy was found to be the cause. Once balanced, their 'bad dreams', minor ailments (attributed to things you have to put up with in life), the reclusiveness, the aggression, and the depression, all faded away within the new white light environment.

A customer of Geomack (15) found that both the children and the family pets were calmer once an Energia unit (see page 111) had been installed. She wrote:

> My family had the system installed two years ago with great success. My daughter who was eight years old at the time was having a lot of temper tantrums which were alleviated almost immediately.

> The greatest surprise success was with our dogs. The male dog was becoming increasingly anxious and barking continually. The day after the system was installed both dogs slept most of the day. After a few days the whole atmosphere became very relaxed and the male dog no longer appeared as troubled. This was remarked upon by most people who visited the house!

Buildings

Houses may be difficult to sell because of geopathic stress. Some people seem to feel that there is something wrong with the house, although they may not be able to identify what it is. Some people also realise that they have never felt well since they moved into a particular house. Occasionally whole roads can be affected by geopathic stress, so that there is a rapid turn over of owners.

People die, divorce or just move on because they do not feel at home. These streets or houses sometimes get the reputation for being unlucky places to live, but nobody knows why.

Geopathic stress can also affect the fabric of the building itself. Pavements and walls can crack, plaster be damp. In these cases remedial work tends to be mysteriously unsuccessful. Often the area will seem gloomy even when freshly decorated. Light bulbs often blow for no apparent reason, and need to be frequently replaced. Alfred Riggs (32) has written:

> It is also frequently found that, apart from this type of radiation having an association with the development of Cancer, it also damages domestic electrical appliances resulting in many breakdowns. The late Dr. Bill Sutherland measured these lines claiming they produced frequencies in the Ghz range. Such is the close proximity of these bands when two different groups cross within the confines of a house it is often impossible to find a neutral zone where a bed could be usefully relocated. Electric light bulbs in such homes tend to have a short working lifespan.

Accident Black Spots

It is well known that some roads have accident black spots. Often there is an obvious explanation such as poor visibility at a crossroad, but sometimes there is no apparent reason. Cars may have accidents there without any other car involved. Often the driver cannot explain why the accident occurred. Undoubtedly some of these will be freak accidents, but is possible that in some cases geopathic energies temporarily interfere with the driver's concentration or vision, and so lead to the accident.

A report in the UK *Sunday Telegraph* on August 10th 2003 and another in the UK *Times* (2003 exact date unknown) give details of a two-year secret trial that had been carried out at an accident black spot in Austria on the A9 between Übelbach and

Deutschfeistritz. Conventional measures such as resurfacing and warning signs had been tried without any effect. Massive pillars (monoliths) of white quartz were erected on each side of the road to restore the energy lines.

Gerald Knobloch who came up with the idea explained:

> I located various elements that had disrupted the energy flow. There was a river which man had forced to flow against its natural direction, various water sources under the ground and a bridge leading over the motorway.

Over a two-year period the number of otherwise unexplained fatal accidents fell from an average of six a year to zero. Harald Dirnbacher, a highways engineer said:

> We were really sceptical at first and certainly didn't want people to know what we were doing, so we kept it secret.....It was an incredible result and we are now planning to expand it by erecting these monoliths at other accident black spots.

Business Considerations

Geopathic stress does not only affect homes. It may also affect work places. This can lead to employees feeling tired and dissatisfied. These places often have a high turnover of staff. Many of those who do stay may be frequently ill, so that absentee and sickness rates are high.

Firms can spend vast sums of money on trying to find out what is wrong. They may change branch managers, bring in engineers to look at the air conditioning and heating, try different ways of organising the work load, ask consultants to interview the staff in an attempt to improve the situation, but nothing works, and the high turnover, absenteeism and general dissatisfaction continues.

In late 1991 an engineer invited me to visit an office block in the City of London. It was a multi-storey building, and he was concerned about two floors that contained offices and a dealing room floor. I had previously talked to him about my work, and he was interested to see what, if anything, I would deduce from examining this particular office block. Sick building syndrome (see appendix 2) had been mooted as the problem, but no conclusive evidence could be found. There was a high incidence of sickness in the building and also a rather mysterious build up of dust on the computer screens. The air conditioning had been overhauled and the work of the cleaning contractors had been examined, but no reason had been found. Everyone was mystified as to what was the cause of these problems.

When I checked the building, I found a large Z of negative energy running through it. I plotted this on a scale plan of the floor of the building. One of the angles of the Z contained particularly turbulent detrimental energy, located within the dealing room floor. Although the dealing room floor was crowded with dealers, it was very noticeable that throughout the morning I was examining the building neither the engineer nor myself saw a dealer standing in the affected area. Other parts of the Z went through offices, and the personnel officer confirmed that nearly all the sick people were sitting directly on the line. The other angle of the Z occurred in a large open-plan office that was particularly known for its high sickness rate, although I did not know that before I did the analysis. When I pointed out where the line changed direction, one of the senior employees accompanying me suddenly ran out of the room. I spoke privately to her later, and she told me that she sat at that exact spot. She had been suffering from a lot of strange symptoms, but had been too scared of the implications to consult a doctor.

The firm concerned occupied two floors of the building. When the same Z was drawn on the plan for the floor above, it became clear that the sick people were sitting one on top of the other. Although many women were employed in these offices, the incidence of pregnancy appeared to be very low. Also there was a colony of feral cats (see page 21) occupying an area just outside the building, but still directly along the line of the Z.

Unfortunately I was not given the opportunity to make the necessary remedial changes, but this study was mentioned in a 1996 lecture "Sick Building Syndrome Reality Or Myth?" given to the annual meeting of the British Association For The Advancement Of Science by Richard Rooley. Richard is a member of the Royal Academy of Engineering. In this paper he says:

> Separately a dowser [Jane Thurnell-Read] plotted the line of high geopathic stress and the personnel manager plotted the work positions of women with high levels of distress and absenteeism... When put together the correlation is remarkable.

Some time later I gave a lecture on geopathic stress, and I mentioned this particular case without saying which building this was. Afterwards one of the people attending the lecture came up to me and said: "I know which building you were talking about." She went on to explain that she had worked for a firm occupying the fourth floor of the building, and that the sickness incidences followed exactly the same lines. In view of our understanding that geopathic energies come from the earth and travel upwards, it is not surprising that workers on the higher floors were also affected.

Giulia Boden (06) carried out some GS work for a company that produced computer databasing systems. The company employed 70 people at the time and had very detailed sickness and absenteeism records. Giulia was able to show how the GS energy occurred in precisely the areas where employees were most badly affected. As with the previous project, she did not know in advance where these people were. Giulia recommended and helped implement changes:

> The results after three months proved conclusively in the eyes of the company themselves that the survey had been a success in improving conditions for staff; this was borne out by a 5% reduction in staff turn-over, and a reduction in sick leave overall, despite a 15% increase in the number of employees.

Shops may also experience problems, as many people will not want to stay in a shop in a geopathic zone. Customers may be unwilling to stay and browse, leaving quickly without really knowing why. The owner and employees may also suffer from poor health and low morale as a consequence of the geopathic stress. Often these shops will have a series of owners, as new businesses struggle to survive. In some shops geopathic problems are more localised, and it is a particular area that is affected. This is often a 'dead' area from a sales point of view.

Hospitals

Patients in hospital beds where geopathic stress is a problem are likely to suffer more post-operative complications and will take longer to get well. After operations people need all their strength to recover. They need the environment to be as near to ideal as possible, but geopathic stress can undermine their energy and their sleep patterns, so delaying their recovery and hindering their progress.

> Mrs. A. Nielsen, a night nurse [in a hospital], found patients in two beds always needed sleeping tablets. After installing a RadiTech [see page 114] no more sleeping tablets were needed.

Classrooms

Children whose desks happen to be placed over negative energy spots will find it difficult to concentrate in school. They are likely to become distracted and either over-active or lethargic, resulting in poor marks, disruption for other pupils and stress and frustration for the teacher. If a large area of the classroom is affected, many of the children will find it difficult to learn, and some of them are likely to be constantly absent from school with varying health problems. This type of situation may well be blamed on the teacher, with adverse comments being made about the discipline and achievements of the children. Because the teacher would probably be feeling the affects of these negative energy forces, he or she would not be in the best position to cope with the difficulties. Many years ago I worked on a primary school classroom, because both the teacher and some of the children were frequently ill. I spoke to one of the teachers at the school some years later and she told me that there was now no difference between illness levels in that room and in the other rooms in the school.

Animals

Not all life responds to geopathic energies in the same way. Some animals (such as dogs, pigs, cattle and horses) tend not to thrive if they live in a GS area. A dog's favourite sleeping place may be a good indicator of a safe place for a human to sleep. Other animals (such as cats, ants, wasps and beetles) respond in a different manner. For them it is a positive rather than a negative and detrimental force.

I have found that a surprisingly large number of houses where there is high geopathic stress also contain cats, which were once strays, and have subsequently adopted the house. Often the owner will recount how they did not encourage the cat to stay. Some even actively discouraged the cat, but nevertheless it persisted in staying around the house, until it was accepted. It may well be that the cat chooses the house because of its negative earth energies. For cats these energies are clearly not negative.

A client consulted me about various health problems, and I found that geopathic stress was part of the trouble. She did not have a cat, but all the local cats spent a lot of time in her garden. I gave her detailed instructions as to what she needed to do to the house to overcome the GS problems. When I saw her the next time, she remarked that not only was she feeling better, but also that the cats had stopped frequenting her garden. Presumably once the negative energies had been corrected, the cats were no longer attracted to the area.

Horses seem to have the same response as humans to these energies. While I was treating a client for her health problems, she told me about a problem she was having with one of her horses. The horse kept re-absorbing the foetus. This was both distressing and expensive in stud fees. A check of the stable showed that there was high geopathic energy within it, but that some nearby stalls were fine. The horse was moved to another stall and given some minerals as a supplement. This time the mare gave birth to a healthy foal.

Dr Joseph Kopp of Switzerland spent some time looking at how animals are affected by geopathic stress. His initial work was with cows. He looked at the earth energies of 130 barns that had housed sickly cows. In all cases he found that negative energy lines ran beneath the barns, often crossing the exact spot where the cows were tethered.

The Dulwich Health Society (13) sells a device to counteract geopathic stress - the RadiTech (see page 114). In their literature they quote this interesting case:

Peter, Sheffield, milking 130 cows – "My cows' cell count was high and they suffered major health problems including very bad feet. After installing a RadiTech not only did my herds health benefit, the cell count came down and the cows actually produced more milk."

Plants

With plants there is a similar situation to that with animals: some thrive in geopathic areas, while others struggle to live and grow. Sometimes trees grow with gnarled and twisted trunks, or lean in a particular direction, in an attempt to 'avoid' the negative energies. On occasions they refuse to grow at all, and wither and die, even though trees near them are fine. Fruit trees may blossom but not set fruit.

Vivian Klein (22), a GS practitioner based in California, helped a vineyard owner to save some of his vines. In part of the vineyard the vines were sick. The owner was contemplating ripping them out and replanting the area with new vines. Vivian told me:

> I advised him to wait and see what happens when I put him 'on the map' [see page 91] – and lo and behold – those vines recovered and are growing strong again for the last 4 years!

Most trees do not grow well near geopathic energies, although oaks, ash, willows, elder and elm have been reported to thrive in such areas. Christopher Bird in *The Divining Hand* recounts a study showing that apple trees develop cancerous growths and that cherries show an abnormal increase in sap. He also writes that plum and pear trees wither if planted over geopathic areas.

I was teaching a group of engineers to dowse for negative energy lines in Hyde Park, a large open area in central London. One of the engineers became very excited when he was able to trace a straight negative earth energy line with his dowsing rods. He was busy looking at his rods and the ground, but I suggested he look up and follow the line with his eye into the distance. As he looked, he became even more excited – all the trees planted close to that line were growing at odd angles bending away from it. Because this is such an open space this could not have come about because of the effect of shade. Neither are severe prevailing winds an issue here. Some of the trees also showed diseased nodules.

Certain plants may not grow at all well in a particular garden in spite of what appear to be textbook conditions for them. A plant may not thrive even though all the growing conditions are right. On being moved to a different spot, even though all the growing conditions appear to remain the same, it suddenly starts to grow and blossom. Plants such as roses, azaleas, privet and celery are believed to not like geopathic stress, but asparagus and mushrooms respond with increased growth and vigour.

Taking into account what should grow well in an area, and what plants and trees are actually thriving in a garden may well give some clue as to whether or not there is a problem with geopathic stress in the house.

Moulds

As well as looking at cows and geopathic stress Dr. Kopp also did some work with foodstuffs and showed that jam became mouldy faster, and wine soured more quickly when kept above an area of geopathic stress. This research with foodstuffs suggests that the microbes that spoil food proliferate in the presence of detrimental earth energies. It has been suggested that a compost heap *should* be located in a geopathic zone, because the vegetation will rot more quickly and so be available to use in the garden sooner.

*****

It can be seen that geopathic stress can affect all aspects of our lives and also that of many animals and plants. Almost any illness can have a geopathic component, depending on the inter-relation of the different ways in which geopathic stress affects individuals.

CHAPTER 3

ELECTROMAGNETIC ENERGIES OR SUBTLE ENERGIES?

Electromagnetic Energies Or Subtle Energy

In a sense the definition of geopathic stress as negative earth energies fudges an important issue – are these energies electromagnetic in nature or something altogether different, perhaps some phenomenon not yet recognised by conventional science?

Geopathic stress is often described as though it is always electromagnetic, involving the earth's magnetic field or electromagnetic radiation. It may possibly be vibrating at a level beyond the electromagnetic spectrum currently detected and recognised by conventional science and technology. If geopathic energies are part of the electromagnetic spectrum this makes them potentially measurable by scientific equipment. It is simply necessary to develop equipment that is sensitive enough to that part of the spectrum.

Some GS practitioners prefer to view the energies as part of subtle energy. If this is true, the energies are unlikely to be measurable by scientific instruments – even more sensitive ones than are currently available. If these energies are not part of the electromagnetic spectrum, different methods of detection are required.

To complicate matters further some practitioners seem initially to define geopathic stress as an electromagnetic phenomenon, but in their subsequent work they approach it as though it is a subtle energy phenomenon.

This is all very confusing, and may be why some practitioners do not seem to address this question at all. They are happy with a general definition and then focus on the effects on people, buildings, plants and animals, and the necessary remedial work.

The Electromagnetic Spectrum

If some aspects of geopathic stress involve electromagnetic phenomena, they may be a continuation of the known electromagnetic spectrum. Electromagnetic radiation has always been part of man's environment. Cosmic radiation, sunlight and the earth's natural magnetic field are part of this electromagnetic 'soup' we live in. The human species has evolved and developed in harmony with this background energy. In fact, it is essential for health. For example, many medical studies have shown that, without adequate sunlight, people suffer from rickets, as a result of Vitamin D deficiency. During winter some people suffer from depression and lack of energy, and this has now become known as seasonal affective disorder (SAD). Treatment with full spectrum light has been shown to be beneficial, but sunlight with its ultraviolet component can also be a problem, with excess exposure leading to skin cancer.

Sunlight is just a part of the electromagnetic spectrum as are radio waves and microwaves. These waves are a combination of travelling electric and magnetic fields, carrying energy from one place to another, from the source to a receptor. Waves can be seen as travelling packets of energy. Electromagnetic energy is a combination of electrical and magnetic energy. Electromagnetic waves consist of perpendicular coupled electric and magnetic fields that travel through space at the speed of light. These differ from mechanical waves (such as sound, water and so on), which are caused by disturbance in a physical medium (such as water or the string of a musical instrument). Visible light itself is an electromagnetic radiation, part of the electromagnetic spectrum.

The different waves have different wavelengths. Waves with a shorter wavelength have a higher frequency. The whole range of frequencies forms the electromagnetic spectrum.

Different waves also have other differing characteristics. For example, some parts of the spectrum can be seen - the visible light spectrum with which we are all familiar - whereas the rest cannot. We are aware of the infrared energy from a fire or an oven because of the heat that is given out. Modern technology can display waves on a monitor such as an oscilloscope, giving a pictorial representation of their shape. Radio waves can be used to transmit sound and pictures in the form of television.

Each energy type affects people in different ways. For example, gamma rays, which are of very high frequency, are given out by substances such as uranium. These are very dangerous to human beings because they can damage our cells, causing chemical changes. These energies can cause severe illness and even death. However, X-rays, which are somewhat longer, of lower frequency, while also potentially damaging, used in the right way can help save lives.

It seems unlikely that geopathic energies are at a higher frequency than the waves that we know about, because the higher the frequency the more devastating the effect on the human body. For example, gamma rays are more dangerous for us than X-rays. If these energies were beyond gamma rays, they would be extremely dangerous. Even a small exposure would have a significant and noticeable effect. There would simply be no argument about whether geopathic stress is a real phenomenon, because even a minute exposure would lead to devastating damage.

Low Level Electromagnetic Radiation

It is possible that these energies are at a lower frequency, at the other 'end' of the electromagnetic spectrum. There has been a lot of discussion about whether low frequency electromagnetic waves are harmful. Much of this has been in relation to power lines and mobile phones (see appendix 1). Scientific understanding is that the lower the frequency the less harmful the wave, as it has less energy. Yet anyone familiar with the power of homeopathy will find nothing strange in the idea that very low-level electromagnetic changes can cause health problems. Homeopathy uses doses of substances that are too diluted to be assayed by normal means. Homeopaths accept that homeopathic medicines are diluted and diluted to the point where it would be impossible to have some of the original substance in every dose. Many scientists say that as there is no material dose of anything in the tablet, any benefit has to be attributable to the placebo effect. Homeopaths respond that the tablet contains the energetic pattern of the original substance and this works at levels other than that of the physical body. There are now scientific studies showing the efficacy of homeopathy (e.g. *Journal of Alternative and Complementary Medicine* Apr 2001, Vol. 7, No. 2: 149-159 and Feb 2005, Vol. 11, No. 1: 21-27). The general public are also becoming increasingly aware of its benefits not only for adults but also for small babies and animals.

The phenomenon of resonance may be the key to understanding how homeopathy could work at such non-existent physical doses and how geopathic energies can have an effect even at very low electromagnetic frequencies. (See page 72.)

Geopathic Energies & Subtle Energy

Some practitioners believe that some or all of the geopathic energies are not electromagnetic at all, but some other type of energy, usually described as 'subtle energy'.

The Concise Oxford Dictionary defines 'subtle' as:

> ... tenuous or rarefied.... evasive, mysterious, hard to grasp or trace... making fine distinctions.

Most scientists, at the moment, do not recognise these types of energy, nor do they have the means to detect these energies, but this does not mean that they do not exist. In an interesting article in *Scientific American* March 1999 George Musser wrote:

> Astronomers...can't find ninety per cent of the matter in the universe.... Something swirls in the heavens and streams through our bodies without a whisper; it cannot be seen.

He goes on to say that scientists have three different ways of weighing the universe and that:

> ... the discrepancies indicate that the universe is filled with some kind of extraordinary matter.

It may be that some or all of this elusive matter is what is referred to as 'subtle energy'.

Drew Leder discusses subtle energy in an excellent article in the *Journal of Alternative And Complementary Medicine* (Vol 11, Number 5, 2005, pp 923-930). He writes:

> This "energy" does not seem to be the sort of electromagnetic, thermodynamic, or other physical energy referenced by $E=MC^2$. Diverse cultures have formulated detailed accounts of other "subtle" energies.

In their book *Healing Sick Houses* Roy and Ann Procter write:

> Throughout this book the word 'energy' has been used as in earth energy and healing energy etc. This is because of common usage

rather than being scientifically correct. We are not referring to a physical energy such as a force, electrical energy or other such forms. The 'energy' we are concerned with might be better described as 'influence' or 'information'.

If geopathic stress is a subtle energy, it is not surprising that conventional scientific instruments cannot detect it. Some geopathic practitioners do use electromagnetic field devices (EMF meters), because they are often concerned about the effect of electromagnetic pollution as well as geopathic stress. EMF meters measure the electric and magnetic fields radiating from electrical equipment and wiring. Some practitioners do not make it clear to their clients that while this may be valuable and important information in its own right, it is not a measure of geopathic stress.

Inconsistent Results

One of the problems of ascribing subtle energy characteristics to geopathic stress is that subtle energies may be malleable by humans through intention, rituals and so on. If this is true, it is possible that geopathic stress is merely a construct of the human will and intention for it to exist.

Drew Leder (*Journal of Alternative And Complementary Medicine* vol 11, Number 5, 2005, pp 923-930) comments that many cultures have a vivid concept of subtle energy and goes on to say:

> While underlying the material universe, such subtle energies can be directed by conscious intent, altered, and transmitted.

Many people who work in this field or in the field of energy medicine would agree with this. While this sort of thinking chimes with the belief that geopathic energies can be altered by intent or by ritual (see chapter 9), it also brings with it the possibility that these energies are a creation of the human mind:

people believe they exist, so they do. While this may be true in some cases, looking at the evidence in this book suggests that in many cases something is going on that cannot be explained in terms of current scientific knowledge.

If at least some geopathic energies are indeed subtle energies, it may also explain why different practitioners find different problems and suggest different solutions. From a scientific point of view this inconsistency is very damning, but it may be, as Roy and Ann Procter in *Healing Sick Homes* suggest, that the analysis that a practitioner does is "a personal mind tool through which to navigate and access energies". The important thing, as they point out, is that whatever remedial action is suggested proves to be beneficial to the clients:

> They [the practitioners] may be attuned to different aspects of the situation, or be using a different type of visualization as a framework. This is all very confusing, but if the object of achieving beneficial results is realised, no matter.

It may well be that what is 'seen' is a combination of the practitioners energy and intent, and the subtle energies manifesting in that place. The actualization of potential model discussed in chapter 9, gives one framework for understanding how this might work.

Some years ago I tried to teach a friend to dowse using rods. He was not having any success, and I got rather impatient, and said silently: "Come on rods, move!" The rods moved. He was very excited, and I was nonplussed. I did not explain what I had done, but as he walked round the rods moved in synchronicity with my intention. At no point in all this did my friend know what I was thinking. This experience really unnerved me, and I still have no completely satisfactory explanation of how something like this can happen.

Anything that is this operator sensitive would be immediately ruled out by conventional science and medicine. But is it possible that operator-sensitive technology is precisely what is needed in the subtle energy world? Quantum physics shows that the act of measuring something changes it in some way, but is not able to predict in advance what that way will be. It appears that the intervention is random. It may be that intent, and therefore operator sensitivity, provides the purpose that can make the intervention non-random. In this way the practitioner's intent becomes a catalyst for a particular positive outcome.

*****

We clearly have two different views of what these energies are: electromagnetic and subtle energy. These two views reflect very different views about the nature of the world and of reality. Of course, it is possible that some geopathic energies are electromagnetic, whereas others are subtle energy. It may even be that any geopathic energy has both aspects within it – a physical presence and a subtle energy counterpart – and that different practitioners are connecting with different aspects of the same phenomenon. Another possibility is that these energies are neither electromagnetic nor subtle energy, so that none of our current understanding really fits.

.

CHAPTER 4

SOURCES OF GEOPATHIC STRESS

What exactly is the source of these negative energies emanating from the earth? There are several different possibilities. Some of these sources suggest that geopathic stress is an electromagnetic phenomenon, but others suggest that it is part of subtle energy.

The Earth's Magnetic Field

The earth has a natural magnetic field. It acts as though it has a large magnet at its centre. The magnetic field is produced by the molten metals that are found within the earth's core. The rotation of the earth leads to electric currents being created in these metals, thereby producing a magnetic field.

Human beings have evolved with this background magnetic field. They are accustomed to living in its presence. It is thought that birds use the earth's magnetic field for migration purposes, and whales may navigate great distances by monitoring it. There is some natural variation in the earth's static magnetic field brought about by changes in weather conditions. These changes are part of the natural diversity of the earth's magnetic field and so do not appear to cause problems. People are also exposed to time-varying magnetic fields, mainly brought about by changes in the sun's activity, but again this does not seem to have a negative effect on people.

Natural Disturbances to the Earth's Magnetic Field

So, the earth's natural magnetic field is not part of what we mean when we talk about geopathic stress. Natural disturbances to the earth's magnetic field may, however, cause problems. This suggests that geopathic energies are at least in part an electromagnetic phenomenon.

These disturbances may be caused by geological faults, underground ore masses and underground water, particularly running water. These sorts of disturbances are relatively stable, although earthquakes and the slow erosion of rock by running underground water can change even these.

Rolf Gordon, the founder of the Dulwich Health Society (13), writes in *Are You Sleeping In A Safe Place?*:

> We have lived with the natural radiations which rise up through the earth's mantle for millions of years. When these vibrations encounter subterranean running water, certain mineral concentrations, fault lines and underground plateaux and cavities, their natural vibrations become distorted and harmful to living organisms.

Rodney Girdlestone in an article entitled 'Are You Building In A Safe Place?' *Caduceus*; Issue No 7, 1989 writes:

> Geopathic zones are characterised by variations in terrestrial magnetism, for the earth's field is not uniform but exhibits many highly localized distortions, some random, some fairly regular. They... occur over geological faults, caves and underground water-courses. These are places where the earth's natural and beneficial field increases or decreases rapidly (there is a high magnetic gradient). Flows of water underground produce the largest effects -- and sewers and drains can be as big a hazard as underground streams.

Jacob Stängle, a German engineer, developed a machine to test for gamma rays. Normally there is a background level of gamma radiation. Stängle invented a machine, a scintillator, to test for variations in this level. He found that underground water veins showed a small increase in the levels of gamma rays at the surface. This increase correlated well with the depth and flow rate of the water. (Christopher Bird, *The Divining Hand*).

Man-Made Disturbances To The Earth's Magnetic Field

Man-made disturbances include mining, foundations for tall buildings, underground transport systems and utilities (sewage, water and so on). These disturbances are increasing as man has made technological advances, changing his use of and relationship to the earth. This again suggests that geopathic stress may be electromagnetic rather than subtle energy.

In many areas mine workings can spread out for several miles beyond the pithead. Public utilities (such as sewage and water mains) while contributing in many ways to improving public health may also cause geopathic energies. Foundations for tall buildings go very deep and may affect geopathic energies, particularly as reinforced concrete contains metal in the form of rods or mesh.

It is, of course, possible that man-made structures and unintentional intervention may improve the situation, by funnelling negative energies away from homes, and so on. Practitioners in this field very rarely hear of such results, because when such a situation occurs people no longer need their help. Obviously, our concern is when the situation is made worse by mankind's activities, because something needs to be done. When things improve without explanation, this may be because of some building work nearby, but we soon tend to take these improvements for granted.

Christopher and Veronika Strong of Stepping Stones (33) describe geopathic stress like this:

> We all need beneficial earth energies for our well-being. However, should this energy be deflected around certain minerals, strata and especially water streams deep in the earth that have been polluted naturally, or contaminated by human activity, this energy is no longer in harmony with our body, but resonating at harmful frequencies. This is called Geopathic Stress.

Unfortunately planners, architects and engineers are not yet sufficiently aware of the need to consider earth energies when locating a building, widening a road, or digging a tunnel.

Electrically Charged Lines

The earth's electromagnetic field comes from deep within the earth, but practitioners are also concerned about naturally occurring grids that they believe cover the surface of the earth. Examples of these are the Hartmann grid (page 41) and the Curry lines (page 40). The way these are described suggests electrical rather than subtle energy phenomena.

The Earth's Subtle Energy Field

Many geopathic practitioners see the earth as having a subtle energy system, just as human beings do. Problems occur when this system is out of balance.

David Furlong in his book *Earth Energies* writes:

> Like us, the Earth has a spectrum of interweaving energies, ranging from the physical level to its spiritual dimensions.

Tom Graves in a paper presented to the Feng Shui Network Annual Conference, in Australia in 1999 said:

...whether or not it's literally true, it's certainly useful, and probably wise, to act as if each place has a mind of its own, a spirit of its own - a genius loci - and choices of its own, too. But personifying a place in this way means that we can converse with it - in imagination, of course, though it may not feel that way - and 'ask' the place for advice, or to 'show' us things we'd otherwise have missed.

Traditional cultures often have elaborate rituals for interacting with the earth and its spiritual nature. Modern thinking tends to scoff at this, seeing it as evidence of a superstitious and uneducated mind. Many geopathic practitioners, however, are convinced that the earth has its own subtle energy system that we ignore at our peril. They believe that interacting and healing the earth is an important part of what they do.

In *Dowsing For Health* Patrick MacManaway writes:

> The first cause of geopathic stress is when we spend extended periods of time in etheric energy fields which, by their nature, are simply not conducive to human health ...... The second cause of geopathic stress is when an otherwise benevolent and healthy energy field becomes stressed and traumatized, and the chi-flow is disturbed, blocked or imbalanced.

And in another part of the same book:

> For the community to be healthy and sustaining, we all need to be in dialogue with the principal tutelary spirit of the landscape. This will guide us in how to form the right relationship with the seen and unseen forces that ultimately act to restore balance to all living systems.

If the earth's self-regulating system is interfered with or overwhelmed, geopathic stress problems are likely to appear. My own research suggests that the earth appears to have 'structures' that regulate the energy flow, removing excess or replenishing energy as necessary (see page 45). When these malfunction in some ways then any geopathic problem becomes more evident.

CHAPTER 5

TYPES OF GEOPATHIC ENERGY

Even if there is little agreement about the exact nature of geopathic energies, there does seem to be more agreement about the different sub-categories. There are many different aspects of energy in its different forms that can be described in scientific terms (frequency, coherence, amplitude, direction, spin, charge and so on), but geopathic energies do not seem to lend themselves to this sort of analysis. If some geopathic energies are subtle energies, it is not surprising that this is so.

Water

Some people interested in geopathic stress concentrate entirely on detecting underground water, although most practitioners recognise that there are many other problems. Water is undoubtedly an important phenomenon but not the only one. It is usually underground water that is the cause of the problem. Surface water, for instance a river or a lake, does not usually seem to cause problems.

In general the faster the water flows, and the greater the volume of water flowing, the greater the geopathic effect. Where water suddenly changes levels, as happens where there are changes in geology, geopathic problems are likely to increase. The problems are likely to be particularly intense at sites over a spot where two underground streams cross, even if there is a considerable depth variation between them.

Underground water does not always cause problems. In his book *Are You Sleeping In A Safe Place?* Rolf Gordon says that problems usually occur when the water is between 60 metres (200 feet) and 90 metres (300 feet) below the surface. He also offers an explanation of how the water has this effect:

> The flow of water rubbing stones etc. creates an electromagnetic field in the opposite direction to the flow of water, which then disturbs the natural vibrations from inner earth going through the water making the vibrations high frequency.

Water that is negative in this way is often referred to as black water. Confusingly, some dowsers use the term 'black water' or 'black streams' to refer to any geopathic energy whether or not it originates with water, so it is important to check what definition any writer or practitioner is using.

Curry Lines

Curry lines are a global grid network of electrically charged lines of natural origin. These lines were first discovered by Dr Manfred Curry and Dr Wittmann. The lines run diagonally (NE to SW and SE to NW). There is some disagreement between different authorities as to how wide apart these lines are, but the consensus seems to be approximately 3 metres (approximately 9 feet) apart, but this can vary. Most practitioners do not see the lines themselves as being a problem. They are concerned with the intersections. Obviously lines that run in this way will have numerous intersecting points. As the lines are electrically charged, the intersecting points are double positives, double negatives or one of each. From his studies Dr Curry felt that the positively charged spots lead to a proliferation of cells, with the possibility of cancerous cell growth, whereas the negatively charged spots could lead to inflammation.

Hartmann Lines

The Hartmann grid also consists of naturally occurring charged lines, running north /south and east/west. It is named after Dr Ernst Hartmann who first described it. Alternate lines are usually positively and negatively charged, so where the N-S and E-W lines cross it is possible to have double positive charges, double negative charges, or one positive and one negative charge. Once again it is the intersections that are seen as being a source of potential problems. The lines are generally regarded as being about 20 centimetres (8 inches) wide and spaced about 2-2.5 metres (6.5 to 8 feet) apart.

Many writers suggest that any intersection within either of these systems is a cause for concern. It is also possible to have spots where the Curry lines and the Hartmann lines cross each other. These spots are generally seen to be more detrimental than a single crossing within the Hartmann or Curry system.

It is difficult to believe that all intersections are harmful, as many nodes would be encountered in the average sized house because of the size of the grids. It is more likely that only certain nodes are a problem. These may have been distorted by other things, such as geological fault lines and underground mining, causing a build up of negative energy there. Another possibility is that they become a problem when a nearby drain (see page 45) is malfunctioning. Rolf Gordon (*Are You Sleeping In A Safe Place?*) does not think that these grids are necessarily harmful either, but believes that they become a problem when geopathic lines cross them.

Schumann Waves

Schumann waves are naturally occurring, beneficial electromagnetic waves which oscillate between the earth and certain layers of the atmosphere. They were first identified in 1952 by Professor W. O. Schumann, a German scientist. He found that these waves have almost the same frequency as brain waves and follow a similar daily pattern. It has been suggested that these waves help regulate the body's internal clock, so affecting sleep patterns, hormonal secretions, the menstrual cycle in women and so on.

Some modern buildings using reinforced concrete, and metal roofs can shield the occupants from these beneficial waves. It may be that part of the reason people suffer from jet lag is that the Schumann waves are much weaker at normal aeroplane altitudes and that the effect is further weakened by the metal fuselage.

Gary Johnson of Subtle Field Technologies (34) uses special L shaped divining rods to assess the Schumann resonance frequency at a site. If the frequencies are distorted, he believes that this is an indication that geopathic stress is probably present in the area under consideration:

> Mrs H's daughter 'A' was undergoing homoeopathic treatment for a variety of symptoms, including: nightmares, behavioural changes, dread of going to school, constant painful sore throats, frequent unwell feelings and listlessness. After several visits to a homoeopath not much improvement was seen, as the initial cause of these symptoms was believed to be the breakdown of her parents' relationship. The case was eventually passed to me after the discovery was made that the child's symptoms had come on within a week of moving into a new house.
>
> Their new home, a three-bedroom terrace house, is situated in an area where I have carried out site surveys on several previous occasions. Geopathic stress had been caused by a geological fault line (common in this area). The fault line ran under approximately

half of the living area, directly beneath the two children's bedrooms (found using divining L rods). Disturbance in the Schumann resonance frequency was practically the same in both of the children's bedrooms (130- 145hertz).

I installed in this bedroom an SFT field resonator [see page 112] that settled the negative energy disturbance. Daughter 'A' has returned to her normal health pattern and no longer complains of the original symptoms.

In the negative effected bedroom the child's homoeopathic remedies were kept on a shelf above the bed. All the remedies tested 'non active', vibrational remedies often take on the distorted energy imprint from a geomagnetic disturbed environment, and become ineffective as medicines.

Black Lines

Black lines are often naturally generated, although quite how this is done is not known. Some, however, may be manifested by malevolent intent or human ignorance. They are usually localised, and do not form a network in the same way that the Hartmann and the Curry lines do. They may well be a subtle energy phenomenon rather than an electromagnetic one. These lines can be straight or curved, at ground level or even above ground level, so that they can be evident on the upper floors of buildings but not on the lower floors. They can also come out of the ground at an angle, so that they miss some rooms entirely or are only present in one upper corner of the room. An unskilled person may miss these lines if they are only looking at the ground to find energy disturbances. There seem to be several different types of black lines. Someone who 'sees' these types of energies described one line as black and depressed, and another as shiny, black, hard and sharp.

Spots And Spirals

Often when we talk about geopathic energies we tend to imply that they are always in lines or streams. Some practitioners in this field, unfortunately, are only able to conceptualise energy in this way. In this case many detrimental energies, such as spots and spirals, may be missed, simply because the only energy which is being investigated is that running in lines. Important energies can unwittingly be excluded because definitions do not include the possibility of finding an energy with those characteristics.

Spirals can have the energy flowing in towards the centre or out towards the periphery. They can be spiralling into the ground or out of it. Although the shape of the spiral is the same, the energy effects are different.

Spirals usually occur in pairs, although only one of the spirals may be found when looking at a particular site because the other is a little way away and not within the perimeter of the site. Spots are usually randomly located on their own. Some practitioners relate spots and spirals to changes in geological structure affecting the electromagnetic field of the earth. Other practitioners describe them in a way that suggests subtle energy phenomena.

Spots and spirals outside the immediate area under investigation can affect the site being investigated, so many practitioners are interested in looking at the area surrounding the building, and not just the building itself.

Energy Clouds Or Fog

An energy cloud or fog seems only to occur inside buildings. They are usually about 3 metres (10 feet) wide. It seems that they occur when energy is trapped within a building in some way, although it can go through walls and ceilings. Perhaps it would be more accurate to describe it as a function of the building and the relationship between walls, so in this sense it does not emanate from the earth. It is caused inadvertently usually by man-made structures not allowing subtle energy to flow adequately, so energy clouds are not found in the open. Psychically an energy cloud has the qualities of an immature energy without clear boundaries, shape or form. One person who can 'see' these things says they look like smoke or fog with a slightly fluttering quality to them. This does not seem to be a particularly detrimental form of energy, probably, at least partially, because they are often located in stairwells and similar places where people do not spend a lot of time.

It has been suggested that people are more likely to trip and have an accident in a stairwell if an energy cloud is located there. Some years ago I was attending a workshop in a building with an energy cloud. One of the participants tripped and had to be taken to hospital as a result of her injuries, which occurred in the stairwell with the energy cloud. Obviously one incident does not prove a theory, but this is yet another possible indicator of the detrimental effect of these energies.

Energy Drains And Switches

Some years ago I discovered a phenomenon which I have named 'energy drain'. When I first discovered it through using kinesiology, I was puzzled as to its exact nature. It was only subsequently that I began to understand more about it. In the locations studied in England and Canada they occur roughly every half-mile (approximately 800 metres) in every direction. They are not necessarily at ground level. The first one I found was in mid air in a room two floors up. I spent some time testing this and other energies that had a similar feel, and eventually came to the conclusion that they are part of the normal structure of things. They are part of the energy system of the planet.

The problem comes when they become 'blocked' in some way, so that energy cannot drain freely through them. It seems that they are essential to the proper dispersal of energy from the physical world into some other dimension in some way that we do not as yet understand. The purpose then of any corrective activity is not to remove or neutralise them.

There are at least two ways in which the drains can become blocked. The first, and most obvious, is if the amount of geopathic energies in the area is so much that the drain becomes 'jammed'. The second way is when the associated 'switch' becomes turned off. Switches are located nearby, usually within 6 metres (20 feet) of the drain itself. It is unclear what the function of these switches is. Why might drains need to be inactivated when they appear to be part of the homeostatic mechanism for the energy system of the planet? Possibly even less clear - who or what would make that decision?

One way in which a switch can be turned off is by placing metal over the switch. This can be done accidentally by putting a washing machine or similar appliance over the switch. There are probably other ways that a switch can be turned off.

Dr Jimmy Scott (16), the founder of health kinesiology, has suggested that energy drains may well act as safety valves, so that a build up of energy can be safely dispersed through these valves. Obviously, if they are not functioning properly they need to be cleared. This allows the energy pressure that has built up to be disbursed, so that the energy drain can take on its normal function again.

The concepts of energy drains and switches seem very different from many of the other geopathic phenomena. We usually want to neutralise, divert or inactivate geopathic energies in some way.

We would rather they were not there. When we consider energy drains we want to restore proper functioning, returning them to full activity rather than removing them altogether.

It may well be that there is a system of drains covering the entire planet. They may be an essential part of the ebb and flow of energy throughout the planet. It seems likely that there are other mechanisms that are like this, forming part of the anatomy of the universe's subtle energy system. If this is the case, these structures too may cause problems when they are not functioning properly. I suspect that this may be a very fruitful area for research in the future.

Vivian Klein (22), a health practitioner and geopathic stress consultant in the USA told me her experience of correcting drains:

> In my own personal experience, once the drain is functioning normally, there is very little GS if any to fix in any particular spot nearby.

> I recently "unblocked" a drain near someone's new home in Canada, and pinpointed a spot in her house where she had to put down an aluminum sheet in her living room and she told me that's the place where all the utilities come into the house from outside. In this case then the extra detail needed was to protect the inhabitants of the house from the EMF's [see appendix 1] coming in - and not necessarily the GS.

Page 116 and 118 includes information on how to correct drains.

Ley Lines

Some people refer to all geopathic energies as ley lines, but this is usually regarded as incorrect. Ley lines are generally recognised as being man-made phenomena, occurring where sacred stones, which have been charged energetically in some way, are laid in a straight line. The ley line appears 'naturally' and spontaneously if at least five energetically charged stones are placed in a line, so that the furthest stones are no more than 25 miles apart. The ley line itself is invisible, and can stretch over many miles, when more than five charged stones are used. Sometimes they are totally above ground.

Some charged stones are spectacular ancient standing stones such as are found in England at Stonehenge and throughout Cornwall. Ancient churches and burial grounds may also be part of a ley line.

Even small stones can be energetically charged either by heating in a fire or by throwing them with considerable force against another rock. The blow or the heat seems to use the energetic charge from the person or people involved, so that the charge does not decay and disappear in the normal way. Lethbridge (see *The Essential T. C. Lethbridge*, edited by Graves and Hoult) and Fidler (*Ley Lines*) give intriguing accounts of charging stones.

Although we do not know about the original events that created ley lines, it is generally felt that ley lines have been made deliberately rather than occurring by accident when people placed the stones there. When I encounter ley lines, they seem to have a very human quality to them, presumably reflecting the character of the people who made them in the first place. It has been suggested that ancient people used these lines as a method of communication. The ley lines may also have been used for delineating pathways and boundaries or for enhancing crop and animal fertility.

Tom Graves has suggested that ancient man was simply amplifying existing earth energies intentionally, and he likened standing stones to a form of acupuncture of the earth (*Needles of Stone Revisited*), whereas most other writers believe that this is not the case. They believe that the makers of the lines were creating the energy lines rather than amplifying existing earth energies.

Ley lines do not necessarily have a negative effect on people exposed to them. It may well be that the ones that do have such an effect have been set up with malicious intent, or else that their initial benign use has in some ways been distorted by later unintentional intervention by man. As Fidler says:

> It has been pointed out that the activities of modern 'civilized' man are fracturing many existing ley lines. One only has to think of the effect of cutting a wide band across country for a modern motorway to realize what damage to the ley system must be constantly taking place. *Ley Lines*

It may be tempting to try to set up ley lines yourself, but Fidler rightly cautions against this:

> As yet we have very little knowledge of the potential power for good or evil of this energy, although there are indications that it can be great. Until such time as we have this knowledge, it is very undesirable to add to or alter the existing system. *Ley Lines*

Mike Rawles (31) has a different concept of ley lines. He acknowledges that ley lines can be man-made but also sees them as being naturally occurring white light earth energy lines:

> The two primary white light 'Earth Energy' influences are Ley (Dragon or Ling Mei) Lines, which carry the Yang [see page 153] and run in straight lines, and the Subterranean Water Lines which carries the Yin and travel in a meandering fashion.

Mike feels that it is possible to have a water line without a ley line, but not the other way round. He believes that it is the edges of the ley lines and water lines that are the problem - inside these lines the health benefits actually increase.

Emotionally Charged Stones

The fact that stones can be energetically charged by hitting them has possibly profound implications for houses built of stone. Do the houses built of dressed stone contain 'something' of the energy of the builder? In one case I found using kinesiology that the stone used to build a client's house appeared in some way to 'contain' a negative emotional vibration, which was affecting her health. On questioning her about this, she said that the builder had gone bankrupt shortly after finishing her house. Of course, he was likely to have known of his financial problems while building her house. Possibly the vibrational quality of his distress was in some way held in the stone of the house as he built it. People living in the house might then have felt this negative vibration in some subtle way. In order for this to happen it is probable that the emotion involved would need to be intense and experienced over a significant period while the house was being built. If this idea is correct, it is important to make sure that the people who build houses are as happy and stress free as possible, or alternatively that the negative energy charge is removed from the building on completion.

A little girl was taken to see health kinesiologist, Pat Ward (38). Her behaviour had changed overnight from being confident and outgoing to clinging and scared, when she started sleeping in a different house. Pat undertook some health kinesiology work with the little girl and also visited the house. Using kinesiology testing she established she needed to put two symbols in the house - one in the room where the little girl slept, and the other in the room directly below. As well as testing where the symbols should go, Pat also tested for the exact design for the symbol. The little girl's behaviour gradually improved. Interestingly the house had been on the market for a number of months but no one had come to see it. The following weekend two couples came. Sceptics will say that this was just coincidence, but people involved in this field know that this sort of 'coincidence' is not uncommon, but as Pat said: "How did they know the energy had changed?"

Pat tested that the house, which was fairly new, had been built on land that had been a slaughterhouse many years ago. Once again this points to the earth 'holding' negative emotions to the detriment of people associated with the place sometimes many years later.

The Paranormal

No discussion of geopathic energies would be complete without a consideration of the paranormal. There is much debate as to what exactly paranormal phenomena are, and whether such things even exist outside some rather hysterical or susceptible people's imaginings.

If, as seems likely, strong thought forms can in some way become attached to buildings, then this may be an explanation for ghosts and so on. Traumatic events, such as a sudden and violent death, may have generated such intense emotions in the person experiencing them that the energy vibration of these thoughts and feelings become imprinted in some way on the building, surviving long after their death. In certain circumstances these thought forms could become re-energised so that 'ghosts' appear in a paranormal 'video'.

It has also been suggested that when a person dies suddenly or very violently, the etheric body (see page 69) may in some sense be 'left behind'. Roy and Ann Procter in their book *Healing Sick Houses* refer to some of the paranormal 'presences' as:

> ... discarnate beings, by which we mean the souls, or non-physical enduring aspects of people who are now dead or have passed on.

Because of the different forms which paranormal phenomena take, it is likely that there is not one single explanation for the exact mechanism of their activity. Whatever the origins of paranormal happenings, it is clear that some people react to them in an adverse way. Various techniques have been used to clear these energies. It is interesting that most of these techniques (such as exorcism) also involve thought forms. It may well be that a strongly positive thought form is imposed on the negative thought form, causing the effect of the negative to be cancelled out.

Mike and Maureen Rawles of Dragonstone (31) work together to deal with GS problems for clients. They have been working with earth energies for 15 years, and geopathic stress problems for the last eight years. Mike told me that in the last couple of years they have begun to realise that one of the biggest problems is the association between 'negative energy areas' (GS) and 'entity energy'. They believe that the entity will feed 50% on the person's energy and 50% on earth energy. If people experience depression, irrational anger and/or reclusiveness, there is likely to be negative entity energy within the house, associated with the negative earth energy that the entity feeds on.

Mike told me that these entity energies are 'not just a cloud of nebulous energy - but something physical enough that it can throttle you'. They have found that occasionally when they are engaged to work on a geopathic stress problem for a client, both the client and they themselves can experience attacks from these entities. Removing all the negative earth energy will, in Mike and Maureen's experience, remove the negative entities, because the entity is no longer being fed by the geopathic energies. Where some but not all of negative earth energies are removed, the inhabitants of the building can be under greater attack as the entity will try to feed off their energy to replace the missing geopathic energy. They see space clearing techniques as being only temporarily effective.

Mike emphasised to me that it is important for this reason that people only tackle geopathic problems when they are sufficiently experienced. They gave me this example from their casebook:

> The lady of the house was suffering extremely disturbed sleep patterns (basically insomnia, and depression), resulting in her visiting a natural therapist. The therapist's resulting recommendation brought Dragonstone to the house. The remote map dowsing showed a 'complex' black water system, which was confirmed on-site, enabling negative energies to co-exist with the house's occupants. The 'balancing' which took more than one visit to finally achieve, brought with it the white light energy, displacing the negative, and returning her to normal sleep patterns. However in the interim period, those in the house actually felt worse, due to the major negative earth energy 'reduction', causing an 'increased' requirement for the negative entity energy to draw energy from them.

Geopathic stress consultant Giulia Boden (06) also believes that it is important to look at the paranormal and geopathic stress together. She told me:

> My experience has been that when clearing entities from a property, they will return if the GS is not then very quickly addressed. The GS provides them with something like a runway straight back into the home.

Tony G. Mills of Applied Energetic Wisdom (03) has also found that certain entities can influence the findings. He says:

> Entities are inappropriate or discordant energies that attach themselves to individuals and buildings. They can confuse the signal when dowsing for GS, sometimes even to the extent of indicating that there is no GS. I test for these inappropriate energies and proceeds to address these entities with the help of the group field; by using certain commands and feeding energy into the field, thus returning these entities to Source.

When I visited Auschwitz and Birkenau I expected to experience at a subtle energy level some of the horror of these two places, which epitomise evil for so many people. I was surprised that I had no sense of the gruesomeness of the place at that level, although emotionally and intellectually I was very aware of it. It may be that subconsciously I was protecting myself from this. Another possibility is that so many people have been to these places with love in their heart for those who suffered and died there that this has neutralised the hatred and evil.

******

Although these different types of geopathic energies have been looked at separately, it is possible to have several of them together interacting and effecting each other and generally making things worse than the sum of the individual energies present.

Unfortunately, geopathic energies do not in general cancel each other out. Instead they tend to exacerbate each other. It is common to have several different types of detrimental energies present in a building. Where several energies overlap, the situation can be quite complex and make an understanding of the problem more difficult. Fortunately it is usually better to consider the whole picture rather than looking at and correcting individual geopathic energies.

It is very difficult to convey a full understanding in words of the characteristics and feel of the different types of geopathic energies. For people who want to work in this field, it is best to develop an awareness of them under the guidance of an experienced and knowledgeable practitioner.

CHAPTER 6

HOW GEOPATHIC STRESS AFFECTS
THE BODY

As with other aspects of geopathic stress, there are many different views as to how these energies have their effect, so this cannot be a totally comprehensive look at all the different theories.

Two Broad Approaches

Our understanding of the mechanisms involved in the damage caused by geopathic energies is at the moment speculative. People working in this field have proposed many different theories, but as yet there is no consensus. It is likely that there are several different mechanisms involved. The theories fall into two broadly different camps. One set of theories sees geopathic stress affecting the body through physical systems. The other approach sees the effect as coming through the subtle energy system of the body.

Medical Models Of Illness

Many people see viruses, bacteria and other foreign agents as being responsible for illnesses; drugs and surgical intervention are seen as being the cure. However, we are all constantly exposed to a wide assortment of hostile organisms, but we do not become ill all the time. If germs *caused* illness, every time we were exposed to a germ we would become ill. This is clearly not the case. The simple answer is that the body can resist most organisms unless and until it is in some way weakened by other factors. One such factor is stress. Some people undoubtedly have inherited problems. For instance, medical evidence clearly shows that both asthma and eczema runs in families, but even here many sufferers know that any form of stress will make their symptoms worse. Before examinations or when general pollution levels are high or when there are financial worries, sufferers will often report that their symptoms are worse. Stress in any of its many forms will exacerbate any situation making the individual more prone to illness.

Overall Stress

The body has a general adaptation to stress, named the general adaptation syndrome (GAS) by Dr Hans Selye, one of the leading authorities in this field. Under stress of *any* kind the physical body shows a specific response. It does not matter whether the stress is emotional (e.g. a fight with a loved one), financial (e.g. loss of a job) or physical (e.g. lack of sleep or working in an environment which is consistently too cold or too hot), the physical response from the body is the same. Hormones control the body's response, and a wide-ranging set of changes occurs. The hypothalamus monitors the physical body. Through its connection to the cerebral cortex it also keeps a check on an individual's psychological state. It initiates the changes necessary to counteract the stress by instructing the pituitary gland that then instructs the adrenal glands on which hormones to release.

There are two parts to this reaction: the alarm reaction and the resistance reaction. The alarm reaction is commonly referred to as the fight-or-flight response, because it initiates the bodily changes necessary to help us successfully run away or fight. The brain becomes very alert, blood pressure increases, breathing quickens and digestion (temporarily unimportant) is slowed.

The second part of the GAS is the resistance reaction. This is slower to start and is more long lasting in its effect than the alarm reaction. In this phase water is retained to help conserve body fluids in case there has been severe bleeding. Blood vessels become more constricted to minimise any bleeding. The hormone cortisol reduces inflammation to prevent it becoming disruptive rather than helpful.

These changes help the body to recover from any physical damage that may have occurred. If the stress continues, however, the body is permanently in a state of apprehension and tension. Gradually the body becomes more and more debilitated by the on-going effect of the stress and less and less able to handle it constructively. The person becomes ill. Blood pressure may remain inappropriately raised. Excess acid may be produced by the stomach leading to stomach ulcers. Decreased activity by white blood cells will lead to less effective resistance to viruses and bacteria. The person may have difficulty sleeping, as the body is on continuous alert. In this situation the body is prone to develop new and more serious problems as overall health becomes undermined. Reduced resistance leads to more frequent infections that further undermine the body, causing a downward spiral of further illness and further debilitation.

The idea of stress as a major factor in ill health is becoming more widely accepted, but the true range of possible stressors is not well recognised. Geopathic stress is one such stress, which is usually ignored because people are totally unaware of its presence.

Geopathic stress is usually a chronic stress with exposure occurring every day often for long hours as a person sleeps in a bed or sits in a chair above negative earth energies. The body is constantly fighting to cope with this on-going stress, producing large quantities of the stress hormones. So geopathic stress can have a general debilitating effect on the body, leaving it open to being more easily affected by bacteria and viruses. Because the body is coping with the effects of geopathic stress it has fewer resources to cope with other eventualities.

This does not mean that geopathic stress necessarily *causes* illness, but rather that by weakening the body it provides a fertile ground in which ill health can flourish. With the debilitating and insidious effects of GS the body becomes weakened and so becomes more susceptible to illness of one kind or another. Its defence mechanisms are less able to resist viruses, bacteria, mould spores, atmospheric pollution and so on. It is the interaction of the two, a body weakened by geopathic stress and a microbe or some other stress, which together cause the problem.

The Body's Electrical System

As well as being generally stressful, geopathic stress could work by affecting the body's own electrical system.

The correct functioning of the body involves many electrical processes. Our brains, governing so much within our body, are basically electrical. Brain waves are electrical signals with frequencies ranging from 0.5 to 60 Hz, which can be detected via electrodes attached to the scalp. Alpha waves with frequencies between 8 and 13 Hz are emitted when the brain is at rest. The nervous system uses electrical impulses that travel along the neurons to send messages throughout the body. Nerves and muscles are stimulated electrically: we are able to move our arms and legs because electrical messages are sent from our brains, via our nerves to our muscles. Even dreaming involves electrical activity within the brain. The heart generates the largest electromagnetic field in the body. When our hearts beat, they produce small electrical pulses.

Medical technology can use this electrical activity to diagnose some serious illnesses. Electrocardiograms (ECG) record the electrical impulses that precede the contraction of the heart, and electroencephalograms (EEG) record the small electrical impulses produced by brain activity.

All body fluids are excellent electrical conductors, as are our tissues. They have to be in order to allow the nerve messages, which are small bursts of electrical activity, to flow freely from the brain. It may well be that this internal electrical activity and the conductivity of tissues make us more susceptible to external electrical and magnetic forces.

External electromagnetic fields can cause interference with television and radio reception, so it may be possible that it can also affect the workings of the human brain in some way. Disturbances in the outer magnetic field by geopathic energies could disturb our own inner electrical and magnetic processes, leading to illness and unhappiness.

The *Taipei Times* reported on March 20th 2005 that the Japanese company NTT had developed RedTacton technology:

> … which it claims can send data over the surface of the skin at speeds of up to 2Mbps -- equivalent to a fast broadband data connection…….. it makes use of the minute electric field that occurs naturally on the surface of every human body

This technology could enable MP3 players and similar to operate without wires, allowing people to download pictures from a camera to a PC without any physical contact between the two. It would also be possible to exchange digital data with another person just by touching them. The inventors believe this will give a more secure digital transmission system than wireless technology does.

Peter Rivett in a short article in the Wessex Cancer Help Centre newsletter (June 1994) offers this possibility:

> The effect of geopathic stress shows up in the distortion of brain rhythms. The alpha brain rhythm increases to about 15 herg (sic) and the corresponding beta rhythm to about 30 herg -- getting closer to the 50 hg (sic) magnetic field generated by our power supply system. Geopathic stress appears to affect the body's housekeeping in the production of new cells and the immune system is weakened. Many affected people complain of not getting a good night's rest and of not having much energy. Because their immune system is below par they are hostage to ill health.

Dr C. W. Smith (*International Industrial Biotechnology Journal*, April 1986) explains how some allergically sensitive people emit an electromagnetic signal at a level that can cause interference with electrical and electronic equipment. This signal can be demonstrated by getting the sensitive person to hold a plastic-cased tape recorder while it is running, but without a microphone in use. A variety of different sounds have been recorded in this way, some of them akin to those elicited from some types of electrical fish.

A study by E R Moraes et al *Physiological Measurement* 2003 24 91-106 showed that detection of changes in the electrical activity of the human stomach, which normally shows a frequency of about 0.05 Hz, could be used as a good non-invasive predictor of gastric disorders.

Pacemakers are designed to counteract erratic electrical signals that cause the heart to beat irregularly. On December 14th 2004 *Scientific American* reported that scientists had managed to culture rat heart cells. Researchers have been able to produce body cells for some time, but heart cells have been elusive, as they tended to lose their shape and stop functioning properly. This group of scientists immersed rat heart cells in a nutrient bath and applied an electrical current to mimic the heartbeat. After eight days single cells had become mature heart cells.

In recent years there has been much scientific interest in biophotons – photons of light emitted by the body. This has also been picked up by people with an interest in metaphysics and complementary therapy. The entry for 'biophotons' retrieved on April 3rd 2006 from Wikipedia, the online free encyclopaedia, says:

> One of the interesting features of biophotons is the enormous amount of interest they have stimulated in diverse fields, including Eastern medicine, acupuncture, martial arts, biophysics, biology, chemistry, theology, theosophy, etc. For example, some have claimed that one might be able to associate "biophotons" with Qi [Chi], a mystical energy source within living beings posited by some Eastern medicine traditions and new-age religions. Research has not yet provided means by which the existence of Qi might possibly be tested, however. It is thus regarded by many as a purely metaphysical construct. Others have postulated that these emissions are related to consciousness.

Marius Hossu and Ronald Rupert describe a pilot study in the *Journal of Alternative And Complementary Medicine* (Volume 12, Number 2, 2006, pp119-124), which showed that chiropractic intervention resulted in changes to biophoton emissions (BPE). Biophoton emissions are correlated with important biological processes such as cell metabolism and nerve activity, so any change in BPE has to be seen as being potentially significant.

Internal Magnets

Jon Dobson and Paola Grassi in the *Brain Research Bulletin* 1996, 39: 255-259 report on a carefully controlled study to show that magnetite was present in normal human brains. There has been speculation that this magnetite may serve a specific function, such as determining location in relation to magnetic poles, but there is no obvious mechanism for this.

In the *International Journal of Alternative and Complementary Medicine* (January 1993) Steve Eabry reviewed research that had found magnetite present in a range of organisms, including humans. Magnetite is an iron ore and is naturally magnetic. It is also called lodestone and was used by sailors to help them navigate. A piece of magnetite was floated on wood in water and, as one end always pointed north, the ship's course could be charted from this. Magnetite has been found in both the adrenal glands and the brains of human beings. It has not as yet been established what role, if any, this serves. However, this would begin to suggest yet another mechanism by which human health could be affected by geopathic stress. The magnetite could be part of the message system of the body. Eabry says:

> It must be recognised that here we have a system continually tuned into very low level magnetic fields, a sensitive receiver looking for information to pass on and utilise throughout the organism. Many, many tiny magnets throughout our brain, ethmoid bone and adrenals, looking for a DC (steady) signal, but instead being twitched by a 60 Hz (60 times a second) signal. It seems obvious that such interference from low strength, man-made fields (that is, at or less than the geomagnetic field or biologically generated field strengths) would be received by this system and would confuse it such that detrimental biological effects would be expected.

Although Eabry is talking about man-made electromagnetic fields (see appendix 1), this could also apply to geopathic energies.

William Philpott, in an article in *International Journal of Alternative and Complementary Medicine* (July 1992), explains how 'there is clinical evidence justifying the conclusion that a negative magnetic field keeps the pH buffer system intact'. This suggests that it is possibly an internal magnetic mechanism that allows our bodies to maintain the correct acid-alkaline balance, which is so important to our well-being. If this is so, it is possible that this delicate mechanism could be upset by external electromagnetic influences, including geopathic energies. In this article Philpott also describes some interesting case studies using magnets to heal, particularly in diabetes. This shows how magnetic forces can be used to affect changes within the body. In this case the changes are, of course, beneficial.

As well as internal magnets, there is some evidence that organisms can be sensitive to low levels of magnetism. As Paul Devereux writes in *Places of Power*:

> It is now known, after a long period of scientific disbelief, that a whole variety of living systems can be sensitive to low levels of magnetism. .... Researchers have found that bacteria can respond to the North Pole or to a magnet moved around them.... Other creatures scientifically tested and found to possess magnetic sensitivity include algae, crabs, salmon, honey bees, salamanders, robins, mice... The list of lifeforms sensitive to subtle levels of magnetism is now very long..... If other organisms can detect magnetism, what about human beings?

Subtle Energy Vulnerability

Interference with the body at a physical level is one possible way in which geopathic energies can have their effect, but another is through the subtle energy system. If this is the case, it is likely to be through damaging the etheric body (see page 69) and the charkas (page 71). This could lead to faulty information being fed to the physical body. It could also mean that ch'i energy does not correctly feed and nourish the physical tissues. Internal subtle energies and the external subtle energies (such as geopathic stress) are seen to share many of the same characteristics.

In the West when we refer to a person having' energy' we mean that they are vigorous and active; we are referring to a physical characteristic. In physics the term energy has a specific meaning: energy is defined as the capacity to do work. Work also has a specific meaning: work is done when a force moves. When work is done on an object, the object gains energy and the source of the work loses energy. Energy exists in many different forms, and it can change from one form to another, e.g. food is an energy source that is changed into physical energy within the body.

We tend to see the physical world as being made up of solid objects, but in reality even solid objects have spaces within them. There are gaps within and between the molecules that make up physical shapes. Atoms themselves are made up of apparently empty space. The concept of molecules and atoms paints a very different picture of the universe from the one we see in our every day world. Molecules and atoms move in ways that we cannot observe with our eyes, but, nonetheless, this movement is real. Subtle energy is seen as existing within and beyond normal matter, forming a blueprint for physical reality. This subtle energy blueprint could well be the mechanism through which the body knows exactly how to grow, so that arms end up the same length and the body repairs itself when injured. John Davidson in his book *Radiation* writes:

> ...subtle energy is the 'ghost'-energy from which physical matter is derived.....In our environment, the harmony or disharmony within subtle energy and the sub-atomic energy patterns, gives rise to the experience of good or bad atmospheres or vibrations....... the disharmonizing of energy fields can ....take place from within-out, as well as from without-in.

Ch'i

The concept of the individual having an energy system is well established in Chinese medicine, where the concept of acupuncture meridians illustrates one aspect of this. In Chinese medicine the basic belief is that a person's health and susceptibility to disease is determined by the health of this subtle energy system. Any damage to this system will ultimately result in damage to the physical body. Many of the alternative and complementary therapies now becoming increasingly popular also use this model for their basic understanding of the disease process.

In this view there is a subtle energy pervading the whole universe, including human beings. This energy is known as ch'i (also spelt chi, ki and qi) in traditional Chinese thought. In Hindu terminology it is called 'prana', and most Western writers refer to it as the 'life force' or 'vital energy'. This energy is seen as being vital for our health and well-being.

All of these ideas suggest that there is something filling the space between physical bodies, or, at the very least, that connections can be made across this emptiness and some sort of 'energy' experienced. David Tansley in *Radionics Interface with the Ether Fields* referred to this as 'the formative matrix' and as the 'energy field giving birth to matter'.

Barbara Ann Brennan, a clairvoyant, writes:

> I discovered that everything has an energy field around it that looks somewhat like the light from a candle. I also began to notice that everything was connected by these energy fields, that no space existed without an energy field. Everything, including me, was living in a sea of energy. *Hands of Light*

Every day experiences can go some way to supporting this too. Think about the effect some people can have on you when they enter the room. Sometimes their presence and energy (for good or ill) goes before them. They are in some sense 'bigger' than their physical body. You are aware of them even before you see them. We have all had the feeling that someone is looking at us and turned to find that this is indeed true. Although we have not even glimpsed them, their concentration on us causes us to turn and see them. In some way the fact that they are looking at us or thinking about us conveys itself to us even though they are not in view.

It is difficult to say what part of us does this sensing, but these instances show that we do sense something beyond physical bodies and beyond what our 'normal' senses can process. Similarly most of us have had the experience of thinking about someone, or deciding to ring a particular person, only to have a phone call immediately from that same person. We often put these events down to coincidence, but for some people it seems to be a very frequent 'coincidence'. There seems to be some link between us and other people, particularly those we love and care about.

Ch'i energy is seen as being intrinsic to the universe: without it there could be no life, although the exact nature of this is not universally agreed. Wikepedia the open access, online encyclopaedia explains:

> Although the concept of qi has been very important within all Chinese philosophies, their descriptions of qi have been varied and conflicting.... One significant difference has been the question of whether qi exists as a force separate from matter, if qi arises from matter, or if matter arises from qi. Some Buddhists and Taoists have tended toward the second belief, with some Buddhists in particular tending to believe that matter is an illusion. By contrast, the Neo-Confucians criticized the notion that qi exists separate from matter, and viewed qi as arising from the properties of matter. [Retrieved 12 May 2006]

Richard Gerber in *Vibrational Medicine* writes:

> ... this peculiar type of environmental subtle energy may have partial origin in solar radiation outside the recognised electromagnetic window of visible light.

Dr Julian Kenyon in an article in the *International Journal of Alternative and Complementary Medicine* (January 1994) describes various types of apparatus used to measure different aspects of the subtle energy system. From this he concludes that ch'i is:

> … related to electrical energy but there are other aspects of Chi which do not seem to relate to electro magnetism as we understand it at the present time.

We are not aware of ch'i itself, because the energy is so perfectly balanced. Ch'i energy has been likened to an isometric exercise. Two equal forces opposing each other give the impression of nothing happening. Neither are we aware of the mechanisms by which we absorb it. Some ch'i energy is absorbed from physical substances: the air, water, food and sunlight, but more is absorbed directly from the universal supply of this energy.

Part of the role of ch'i within the body seems to be to provide information to cells and between cells. This is information over and beyond the information supplied through the nerves and the hormone system. Disease can be seen as a sign that the flow of ch'i is in some way faulty or unbalanced.

Kirlian photography claims to produce images of subtle energy, by photographing objects with special apparatus. Also known as electrography, it was developed in Russia by Semyon Kirlian. Photographs are taken in the presence of a high frequency, high voltage, low amperage electrical field. This produces a halo around the object that is said to represent the energy field of the plant, animal or person who has been photographed. Kirlian photography shows how different halos are generated by organic and non-organic vegetables and by sick and healthy people. It also claims to be able to provide information about a person's physical and emotional health based on photographs of the hands.

The Acupuncture Meridians

The subtle energy system is partially based on the meridians. There are fourteen major meridians, mainly running skin deep over the head, torso and limbs. The meridians are mainly bilateral, running as mirror images on both sides of the body. It is believed that ch'i enters the body and is distributed throughout the body through the meridians.

These meridians are named after specific organs (e.g. the liver meridian, the small intestine meridian), but are not necessarily on 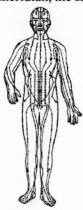 or near the named organ. For example, the lung meridian runs down the inner arm to the thumb. The acupuncture meridians can relate directly to the health of the internal organ associated with it. The meridians are paired together. Each pair consists of a yang meridian and a yin meridian. Yang meridians reflect qualities such as expansiveness, dryness, masculinity, lightness, heat and hollowness. Yin meridians reflect qualities of femininity, receptivity, darkness, coolness and solidity. The yang meridian needs its paired yin meridian for its completion, so, for example, the large intestine is paired with the yin meridian of the lung. (See appendix 3 for a more detailed explanation of the terms 'yin and 'yang'.)

The meridians form part of the inter-face between the physical and etheric bodies. Acupuncture points lie along these meridians and it is these that are needled during acupuncture treatment. The aim of this is to balance the flow of energy within the meridians. Skilled practitioners can 'feel' the location of these points. For a long time the power of acupuncture was dismissed by Western medicine, because acupuncture theory did not fit with the medical understanding of how the body functions. However, gradually some doctors began to find that acupuncture could work for pain relief. As the body of evidence for the success of acupuncture with adults, babies and animals mounted, medical researchers began to consider the possibility of these subtle energy concepts such as meridians more carefully, although many feel acupuncture works through the nervous system in some way. In fact, the reality of meridians and acupuncture points is now beginning to be documented using radioactive tracer isotopes and sensitive electronic equipment. This suggests a real physical presence for the meridians.

The Subtle Bodies

Everyone recognises that human beings are not just physical bodies, but many traditions and therapies have a complex theory of subtle bodies to explain this additional 'something'. There is some disagreement about how many subtle bodies there are and what they are called. Most writers on this subject accept that, as well as there being a physical body, there is also an etheric body, an astral or emotional body, one or more mental bodies and a spiritual body. Many systems include additional bodies.

The physical body is the material body that we can see, composed of atoms and molecules, obeying the laws of physics, chemistry and biology. The etheric body is said to contain the blueprint for the physical body, determining how the foetus develops and how the body repairs itself when damaged. As the embryo develops, the single original cell divides and replicates itself many times. In some way, not yet fully understood by science, these cells eventually become specialist cells with a specific function in a particular part of the body. Richard Gerber in *Vibrational Medicine* writes:

> This field or 'etheric body' is a holographic energy template that carries coded information for the spatial organization of the fetus as well as a roadmap for cellular repair in the event of damage to the developing organism.

The emotional body is the centre for emotions and is also where the 'atmosphere' around people is generated. The mental body or bodies is the source of thought, both practical day-to-day thought and abstract philosophical thought. The spiritual body contains the sense of something other than the human world, something that some people would call 'the divine'.

Many diagrams of subtle bodies show the higher bodies surrounding the lower bodies, but this is probably far from the truth. All the bodies inter-penetrate each other and are inter-connected in myriads of different ways, which are impossible to show adequately via a diagram. They should be viewed much more as an inter-connecting web, rather than as layers in an onion or separate entities. Each subtle body is seen as having its own vibrational rate. The physical body is visible precisely because it has a low vibrational rate whereas the spiritual body cannot be seen because its vibrational rate is so high. The terms 'higher' and 'lower' are often used for these bodies, with the physical body being the lowest and the spiritual body the highest. This is unfortunate terminology, because it suggests that the physical body is in some way inferior to the other bodies. All of the different bodies need to function and inter-relate for a human being to be healthy and happy.

We tend to think of our bodies as being static once fully developed, except perhaps for the changes which take place with age. Yet the body is continually renewing itself. The physical body you have now does not contain any atoms or molecules that are the same as those that were 'you' fifteen years ago. The molecules are so slowly replaced that we have the illusion that our eyes and hands and face and internal organs are the ones we had all those years ago: after all they look the same apart from signs of ageing. There is some observable evidence for this process in the way in which hair and nails grow, and skin flakes and peels. As Deepak Chopra writes in *Quantum Healing:*

All of us are much more like a river than anything frozen in time and space. If you could see your body as it really is, you would never see it the same twice. Ninety-eight per cent of the atoms in your body were not there a year ago.

Chopra goes on to give figures for the rate at which various parts of the body change. He writes that the skin is replaced within a month, the stomach lining every four days, the liver is completely renewed every six weeks.

Alternative therapists believe that the etheric body provides the blueprint for the physical body. This allows the body to replicate itself continually. This constant renewal of the body gives the possibility for profound healing, but it also gives the possibility for damage and harm to come to it. One possibility is that geopathic energies interrupt in some way this process of renovation and renewal that carries on all the time unseen by us and without our conscious awareness. If this is the case, it is very likely that exposure to geopathic stress can lead to illness.

If geopathic energies affect our subtle energy system, it would mean that they are not necessarily processed by the physical body, but directly affect the subtle bodies. The physical body is then affected by its connection and inter-dependence on these other bodies for its overall health. This would, for example, explain the link between geopathic stress and cancer. In cancer rogue cells continue to grow, as the physical body seems to have lost its ability to destroy them. If part of the etheric body's role is to offer a controlling blueprint to the physical body, this blueprint may be damaged by geopathic stress and so contain faulty information.

Chakras

Although the individual subtle bodies have different vibrational rates they have to be connected in some way. This is one of the functions of the chakras. In Sanskrit chakra means 'disk' or 'wheel', which is how the chakras often appear to clairvoyants. Most writers in this field suggest that there are seven major chakras: the base chakra, the abdominal chakra, the solar plexus chakra, the heart chakra, the throat chakra, the brow or third eye chakra and the crown chakra. Each chakra is seen as having particular characteristics (such as emotional qualities, colour, sound, and so on) associated with it. Each chakra is also linked to a particular organ of the endocrine system. So, for instance, the throat chakra is related to the thyroid gland (located in the throat) and is associated with the emotions of shyness and paranoia. The brow chakra is associated with the pituitary gland (the master gland of the hormonal system) and with the emotions of anger and rage.

Chakras connect the different bodies and provide a mechanism whereby the vibrational frequencies of one body can be accepted by another. The chakras are the equivalent of step-down transformers. They change energy from one form to another, thereby allowing interaction between the various subtle bodies. It is likely that these are also damaged by geopathic energies. If this is the case, then some of the essential energy connections between the different bodies may not occur, leading eventually to illness.

Resonance

Geopathic energies may affect specific parts of the body directly by causing damage through resonance. All objects have a natural frequency, which can be set in motion or increased by something nearby which is vibrating at the same frequency or pitch. When this happens we say that the two things resonate. An opera singer can break a glass by singing a note with the same frequency as the glass. The glass will be affected by the note, start to vibrate at the same frequency to such an extent that it will shatter. In the 1940's the Tacoma Bridge in the USA collapsed because a crosswind caused resonant vibrations of the structure, which led to it swinging so much that it broke up.

Resonance is the frequency at which maximum energy transfer takes place. Resonance can be seen in a less spectacular form in every day life: parts of cars rattle when the engine reaches a particular speed, and parts of houses will also rattle when heavy lorries go past. The vibration of one is causing the resonant vibration of the other.

Every organ of the body has its own resonant frequency. Different geopathic energies appear to vibrate at different frequencies giving them their own unique qualities and also their ability to affect human beings. As with the opera singer and the glass, if the GS energy resonates at the same frequency as a body organ then it can damage that organ. The greatest damage occurs when the maximum resonance is being experienced.

*****

As with almost every other aspect of this fascinating subject, it is clear that there is no real consensus on how these energies affect the body. It is likely that there may be several different mechanisms involved.

CHAPTER 7

INDIVIDUAL SENSITIVITY

It is evident that even though geopathic energies may be present in the environment not everyone who is exposed to them necessarily experiences problems. It appears that the relationship between geopathic stress and the individual is not straightforward. There is a glimpse of this in Patrick MacManaway's definition of geopathic stress in his book *Dowsing For Health*:

> Geopathic stress is best considered as a dysfunction in the relationship between person and place.

Giulia Boden (06) told me:

> The energy of the house can in many cases reflect the person's own energy, albeit often in a subtle way, and vice versa; the two energy systems are intrinsically linked, physically, emotionally and spiritually. In this age when we often see our weaknesses mirrored in our relationships with others, our own living spaces are just another sign. How badly we are being affected may well be a message to us to explore within ourselves more deeply, and could have a pivotal effect on our lives.

David Furlong in *Earth Energies* defines geopathic stress as:

> Our response to a natural physical or subtle earth energy pattern which in itself may be neither good nor bad.

Geopathic energies do not affect everyone in the same way. Some people may be severely affected; others may be relatively immune. One person may suffer stomach problems, while another suffers with headaches. There are several possible explanations.

Overall Sensitivity

Undoubtedly some people are generally more sensitive to GS energies regardless of the type or source. It is possible for several people to live in the same house and only one of them to be affected by the geopathic stress. This phenomenon is also found with other types of stress. One person may be able to suffer many emotional traumas and remain in good health, while another will crumble at the first severe emotional problem. Yet a person who cannot cope with emotional distress may be able to continue functioning on very little sleep, for example.

Resonant Frequencies

It is clear that there are many different types of geopathic energies, each with its own characteristics, so that an individual may be sensitive to some of these energies more than others. If the environment has geopathic energies, but not the ones that the individual is sensitive to, geopathic stress will not be experienced.

There also appear to be gender differences in sensitivity. I first got an inkling of this when I was using muscle testing (see page 88) to test a group of people against a specific geopathic energy. Much to my surprise only some of the women reacted to it, and none of the men. When I thought about this further, I realised what the explanation might be. At least some of the damage caused by geopathic energies may be caused through resonance (see page 72). If this particular geopathic energy had a vibrational rate close to that of a female organ, females are more likely to react adversely to that geopathic energy.

Another possibility is that there may be a frequency range for a healthy liver, for example, and that a person with an organ resonating at the exact frequency of the geopathic energy is more affected by the energy transfer than someone whose liver is further away from that exact resonance. Alternatively, if the person already has an unhealthy liver, that could be vibrating at the same frequency as a geopathic energy. In this situation the health of the liver would deteriorate even more, while someone in the same environment but with a healthy liver would be much less affected.

All this, of course, complicates the picture, but also explains why some people can live in a house without any apparent problems, while others are ill.

Patterns Of Use

People's pattern of exposure to geopathic stress may vary even if they live together in the same place. For example, someone who is at home all day in a geopathically stressed house is likely to suffer more than someone else who lives in the house but goes to work in an environment with little GS. In a house where the GS problems are worst in the kitchen, the keen cook may be more affected than other members of the family.

Overload On Particular Body Parts

It may also depend on the parts of the body that are most directly in contact with the geopathic energy. A person can be affected in a particular part of their body because a negative energy line crosses that point while they sleep. When energy lines are plotted through a house, it is interesting to see how often the negative line will be located across the person's bed. Occasionally all of the bed is affected, but sometimes the negative line is more localised, so that the occupant will be exposed to these forces only in a limited part of their body. Frequently the organ or tissues that are the focus of the illness will correspond to this. Kathe Bachler's book *Earth Radiation* documents many examples of this phenomenon.

Christopher Bird in his book *The Divining Hand* quotes the words of Herbert Douglas, an American dowser:

> I thought that the underground veins could be best illustrated if I laid out a series of wooden laths on the bed to show the direction of their flow. When I did this, I asked the person who slept in the bed to lie down in the position they normally assume when falling asleep. Repeatedly, the crossing of the laths indicates precisely where the person is afflicted.

British dowser, Alfred Riggs (32) describes a graphic case study that illustrates this:

> At the Manny Patel Cancer Clinic in Bangor, North Wales, I was called upon to examine the house of one of their patients. It is my standard practice not to have any information related to the house or individual health problems, in order to conduct a blind investigation. In this case, however, I was in receipt of the knowledge that someone living in the house was suffering from Cancer. After dowsing five sleeping sites, I was able to state that the person in question slept on the right hand side of a double bed, and if they slept on their back, the Cancer would be in the area of the left breast, if they slept on their stomach it would be located in the area of the right breast.
>
> A member of the staff who watched me working said: "You have found the right bed and the correct side but the patient sleeps on her back and has the Cancer in her right breast, not the left as you suggest." Arising from this, I was able to state with some confidence that the bed had been moved recently some 8-10 inches to the left. They then consulted a member of the family who confirmed the bed had been moved in order to accommodate a bedside cabinet. When the cabinet was removed we could see the original position of the bed by the imprint left in the carpet. Measuring the leg of bed positions from the centre to centre established it had been moved some 8.5 inches to the left, bringing the crossing point of the lines of radiation in the area of the right breast. It is possible to be this accurate particularly when the lines are a combination of the narrow

bands generated from the underground water movement and geological fault lines.

Some years ago I was involved in a programme for the UK television station Channel 5. I was asked to assess a house from a GS point of view without knowing anything about the inhabitants. I found a negative energy line running across the bottom part of one side of the double bed. I predicted that whoever slept on that side of the bed was likely to suffer with lower back or leg problems. It was subsequently revealed that the husband slept on that side of the bed, and some nights was woken by leg cramps. I also predicted, again correctly, that if someone liked a particular chair in the lounge, they would be likely to suffer with headaches or migraines, particularly as the line was not at ground level but about head height.

Weakest Point

Another possibility is that the geopathic stress is affecting the person's weakest point, so producing illness. If the throat is the weak point, the person is likely to suffer from throat problems, whereas if the stomach is the weakest organ then digestive problems may appear after exposure to negative earth energies. The effect of geopathic stress is to aggravate an underlying weakness in the body.

Using Indices

All this suggests that in assessing geopathic stress problems it is important to consider not only the absolute measure of geopathic stress for a particular site, but also an individual's sensitivity to the range of energies present there, and how much time they spend in any localised areas of stress.

So, for example, you could have four individuals living in the same house over a geopathic 'hot spot'. Two of the people in the house (A and C) are generally well. One person (B) has chronically poor health. The fourth person, D, has health problems, which sometimes clear up when he is away from home for a considerable length of time. At first sight, it might not seem likely that geopathic stress is involved, because not everyone in the house is ill. Understanding that individual susceptibility is important puts a completely different complexion on this. Here is one possible explanation of the different experiences of these four people:

- A is not generally susceptible to geopathic problems, and so has no particular health problems.
- B is severely affected by geopathic stress in general, and suffers with chronic health problems in spite of visiting many conventional and complementary practitioners.
- C is strongly affected by one type of geopathic energy, but it is not found in this locality, and has few health problems.
- D is strongly affected by one type of geopathic energy that is found in the house, and struggles to get well and stay well. D does sometimes feel better when away from the house for a substantial length of time (i.e. when in an environment that has minimal geopathic energy, or energies that he is not sensitive to).

I have, of course, simplified this by excluding any health problems attributable to other reasons. These would make the situation even more complicated. For example, if such factors are included and two more people (E and F) are added to the house:

- E is not generally susceptible to geopathic problems, but has undiagnosed allergies so has a series of health problems.
- F is mildly sensitive to geopathic stress and also eats an

appalling diet, drinks too much alcohol, etc. but at the moment has no obvious health problems. (F is in his 20's and the effects of his unwise life-style are not yet evident.)

When I was an active GS practitioner, I usually used an indexing system to deal with all these different parameters. I first established (using kinesiology – see page 88) an absolute measure of the geopathic energies for the building or area on a scale of 0 to 100. 0 meant that there were no geopathic energies at all, and 100 meant that it would be impossible to make the site more geopathically stressed.

I then established a measure of each individual's sensitivity on a scale of 0 to 100, where 0 indicated the person is not at all sensitive to the geopathic energies present, and 100 indicated that they would die instantly on exposure to them. The scale also took into account how the individual used the area being assessed, so for example if a negative energy line crossed their bed this would rate higher than one in the kitchen, where they spent less time.

I then multiplied the two indices together to give a sensitivity measure for that individual for that property. The answer often seems at first sight alarmingly high, but the maximum is now 10,000 (100 x 100). Fortunately remedial action can usually be taken to reduce this. In my experience the number needs to be below 22 for that person not to have a problem with the energies. This may seem impossible because of the high numbers often involved, but because of the multiplication process, removing small amounts of geopathic energy gives big reductions.

If all the geopathic stress were removed, the figure would now be 0 for everyone's susceptibility. Rechecking the individual's sensitivity index after the remedial work, gives a measure of how successful the work has been at reducing the GS energies that the person experiences as a particular problem. This may be particularly useful if it is not possible for some reason to counteract all the GS energies present. Then I combined the two measures (the new index for the property by the new index for the person) and made sure it was below 22. Ideally, of course, I would want the figure to be zero, but sometimes attaining that level of perfection was extremely difficult and in my experience not always necessary.

CHAPTER 8

DETECTION OF GEOPATHIC STRESS

Most people will need to bring in an experienced practitioner to detect and correct geopathic stress, unless they use one of the proprietary devices on the market (see page 110). Before spending any money it is possible to get some sense of whether pursing this line of enquiry is worthwhile.

D.I.Y. Detection

Once introduced to the concept of geopathic stress, many people find that they can sense where the best place in the house is and, perhaps more importantly, where the worst place is. Many people's pulse rate will increase significantly when they are standing in a geopathic area for a while, so that this can be a useful guide too.

Many small babies seem intuitively to move away from negative energy lines, so if a baby is observed always sleeping at one end of its cot it probably indicates that the cot should be moved towards the preferred end.

Chapter 2 suggests ways in which observing our environment can lead us to suspect geopathic problems. Observing the behaviour of animals can reinforce information gained in other ways. Dogs react in a similar way to human beings to geopathic energies, whereas cats appear to prefer them. This can give important indicators of where any problems are in the property.

Looking at the plants and trees that thrive or fail to thrive could indicate whether a GS practitioner should be brought in. Observing the general environment may suggest that there are likely to be geopathic energies present. Do light bulbs blow frequently? Does electrical machinery fail more than it ought to? Is there a place where people keep tripping or dropping things for no obvious reason?

Persistent damp can be an indication of the presence of geopathic energies. Obviously a lot of damp exists because of poor ventilation, leaking roofs and so on, but if all the obvious structural faults have been corrected and damp still persists, it may well be worth looking at the possibility of a geopathic energy involvement.

Taking all these factors into account can give a good indication of whether involving a GS practitioner is likely to be money well spent.

Calling In An Expert

There are three main methods that practitioners use to assess a property for geopathic stress. Some people can dowse (using rods or pendulums). Others use kinesiology (or muscle testing as it is often known) to track these energies. Some individuals can 'see' or 'sense' these energies.

All of these strategies seem to use what Aubrey Westlake called our 'supersensible sense' (Foreword to David Tansley's book *Radionics Interface with the Ether Fields*).

Dowsing

Dowsing is sometimes also called 'divining'. It is an ancient art that is now enjoying a revival of interest. Dowsing has mistakenly been associated with the occult by many, so that dowsers often do not talk about what they do. You may well know a keen dowser without realising it. However, dowsing is now being viewed more and more as a practical tool. It is being used to detect water for farmers and water boards, and to detect minerals and oil by some exploration companies. Unfortunately this positive use of dowsing is often not widely publicised by the companies involved for fear of ridicule.

Dowsing has been around for a long time. Depictions of people dowsing have been found on Egyptian murals and ancient Chinese statues, but the real documentation of dowsing began with French priests in the seventeenth century. However, much of the knowledge about dowsing is not written down, but is passed on by teaching and demonstration by experienced dowsers.

Dowsers often use pendulums when dealing with individual health problems. The pendulum consists of a weight (usually made from wood, crystal or metal) suspended on the end of a string or thin wire, which the dowser holds between two fingers. The pendulum swings one way for 'yes' and another way for 'no'. The most common response is clockwise for 'yes' and anticlockwise for 'no', but different people get different responses. The important thing when using a pendulum is that the response is consistent: a particular response from the pendulum always meaning 'yes' and another, equally clear response, always meaning 'no'.

Dr Patrick MacManaway in his book *Dowsing For Health* says:

> Dowsing works very simply. We ask a clear and unambiguous question in our mind, to which the answer can only be "Yes" or "no". Having asked the question, we allow the answer to come back

to us from our inner self, using a predetermined code to interpret the movements of the dowsing tool to indicate whether it is a positive or a negative response.

Dowsers generally use a short pendulum or bob. The weight is suspended on a thin cord about 25 cms (8 inches) long. Some dowsers 'ask' for the pendulum to swing in a particular way when they are standing over an area of geopathic stress. Sometimes dowsers carry a 'witness' in their hands while doing this. Some pendulums have a space in the weight to house the witness. A witness is a sample of the thing that the dowser is trying to find. Providing a sample is not a problem when the object of the search is water or a particular metal. However, it becomes more of a problem when the dowser is searching for geopathic energies, although some companies do offer 'witnesses' for different geopathic energies.

Some dowsers use the long pendulum. Here the weight is attached to a much longer cord, often about 100 cms (40 inches) in length. The dowser will adjust the length of the cord according to what he or she is looking for. Considerable work on this was done by T.C. Lethbridge (see *The Essential T. C. Lethbridge*, edited by Graves and Hoult). He found that his long pendulum gyrated in the presence of copper when the length of the cord was 30.5 inches, in the presence of iron when the cord was 32 inches and so on. He also found that the pendulum would react to ideas. Interestingly, silver and the moon both caused a rotation of the pendulum at 30 inches, but the number of rotations would be different depending on which he was thinking about. To the best of my knowledge there are no specific lengths yet established for geopathic energies.

Using a pendulum while walking will often cause a pendulum to sway with the motion of the body, so that any finer movement caused by changing geopathic energies are not so easily observed. For this reason GS practitioners often use rods rather than a pendulum, as this allows them to walk around the building or surroundings without their movement overly influencing the rods. If there is a strong wind, this becomes a problem even for the user of rods, as they can wobble in the wind, giving false readings.

The rods are usually made of metal, although sometimes a forked twig, traditionally made of hazel or willow, is used instead. One reason for using willow was that willow is found near water. As the early dowsers were usually looking for water, they felt that willow had some affinity for it because of its preferred habitat. Learning to use dowsing rods has been described as being like training a pet dog – the rods being the dog. The dowsing rods are 'trained' to cross when the dowser is above the negative energies. Some dowsers train their rods to cross when *their feet* are above the area, whereas others have their rods cross when *the rods* are above the energies. The rods may also be used to point in the direction of flow of an energy or to point out a relevant spot or area.

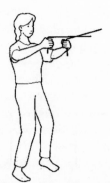

I once had a rather strange experience with dowsing rods when I was in London. I was walking with some other people towards Hyde Park in the centre of London with the intentions of doing some dowsing in the park. I was holding my rods in the normal dowsing position, as I walked along the road. I was not really paying them much attention, because I was talking to the person walking next to me. Abruptly and swiftly the rods moved through 90 degrees. I have never seen rods move so fast and so 'purposefully'. The rods were pointing directly at a building. There was a policeman standing outside the building. I walked over and saw that the building was an embassy. The government of that embassy was involved in an acrimonious dispute with the British government, which believed that it was supporting terrorist activity. Normally when you use dowsing rods you have some intention. For example, you might set out to look for water, geopathic energies or minerals. My intention (but without much focus) had been for the rods to find anything 'interesting' on my walk to the park. My suspicion is that the rods probably picked up the activity of some sort of surveillance equipment. It was certainly an 'interesting' find.

In *The Divining Hand* Christopher Bird explains how Dr Zaboj V. Harvalik, a physicist and scientific advisor to the U.S. Army's Advanced Material Concepts Agency, undertook to find out more about dowsing. He conducted various tests and concluded that the organs in the body responsible for sensing these changes were the adrenal glands and the pineal gland. The stimulus was then transmitted to the brain and back out to the muscles of the arms. He also concluded that almost anyone could be taught to dowse, although many people needed to drink some water before starting to dowse. He also found that many dowsers could activate rods in other people's hands simply by thinking 'exciting thoughts'. (See also page 32.)

There is no totally convincing explanation of *how* dowsing works, but there is more and more evidence that it *does* work. Most authorities on dowsing agree with Harvalik that the dowser picks up minute variations. These variations cause minor changes in muscles including those in the wrists. The rod or pendulum then makes these changes visible to the naked eye, and thereby to the conscious attention of the dowser. A small change in muscle tension becomes a much larger change in the movement of the rod or pendulum. Having said this, dowsing should *feel* as though the rods or pendulum are moving of their own accord and are not being influenced.

This, however, does not explain how many dowsers can work from maps (see page 91). Both Harvalik and Tom Graves recognise that as yet there is no adequate explanation of how map dowsing works, but both believe that there is incontrovertible evidence that it does. Tom Graves points out in his excellent book *The Dowser's Workbook*:

> Dowsing rarely makes sense in theory, but does work surprisingly well in practice if *you* let it work.

His book takes the reader step by step through the procedure of learning how to dowse. It also explains how to make a dowsing rod from two metal coat hangers and how to make a pendulum from a cotton reel or a used AA battery. Dowsing societies such as the British Society of Dowsers (06) also offer short courses in dowsing for anyone interested in learning this fascinating skill. The Society feels that most people can learn the art 'by practice and perseverance', although some people will have a more natural aptitude for it than others.

Kinesiology

Dowsing uses rods or pendulums to amplify the body's response, but kinesiology uses the observable response of a person's muscle or muscles. Kinesiology was developed by Dr George Goodheart, an American chiropractor, in 1964. The discipline originally called kinesiology, used by physiotherapists and others, is concerned with the 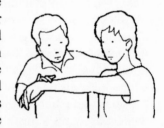 mechanics of movement and the physiological state of the muscles themselves. Kinesiology as developed by Dr Goodheart went beyond this, using the muscle response as an indicator of other aspects of the body's functioning. He discovered that testing muscle response reveals other things about the body. For instance, it can be related to the acupuncture system or to organs of the body. Kinesiology has continued to develop and can be used to treat health problems very successfully. It can also be used to measure geopathic stress.

In kinesiology a muscle response is used for assessment. Usually one of the arm muscles is used for this. At its simplest, muscle testing involves getting the person to hold one of their arms in a particular position. This position is chosen to isolate as far as is possible the action of one muscle, so that any weakness of functioning becomes easily evident. With the client's arm in the correct position, the tester applies gentle pressure on the arm. Under this pressure the arm either locks in position (a positive or 'yes' response) or gives way (a negative or 'no' response). This is not a form of arm wrestling, or designed to test how strong a person is, but is a sensitive test of the muscle response to different stimuli. Both people should use the same amount of resistance each time. Obviously there will be slight variations in the amount of pressure used, but these small variations are within the tolerance for the test when performed by a skilled practitioner.

The kinesiologist will test a client to check out whether geopathic problems are present in their environment and also what they are. They may ask the client to stand in different places on the site and test the muscle response. If the arm gives way, this indicates that the person is in some way stressed by what is happening or where they are standing.

This can be a slow and laborious way to check for geopathic energies, so many kinesiologists will use the on/off response of the muscle, as a yes/no response. The practitioner asks a verbal question, out loud or silently, applies gentle pressure on the test muscle and assesses the response. If the muscle holds, this indicates a 'yes' response. If the muscle is spongy or gives way when tested, this means 'no'. This procedure allows a skilled kinesiologist to ask a series of questions where the answer has to be 'yes' or 'no'. In this way the exact nature of the problem and the remedial action can be established.

Some kinesiologists use self-testing instead. This is a technique where they test one of their own muscles with another muscle (usually those of one finger with another finger, or one hand with the other hand), rather than using a client's muscle.

Sensing the Energies

Both dowsing and kinesiology can be taught to the willing student, but sensing energies is a much more difficult skill to pass on. When you talk to people who can 'see' or 'sense' these energies they often find it difficult to explain how the process happens and what exactly it is that they see. They may say that the air appears less clear, less vibrant or denser in areas of geopathic stress. They may say some geopathic energies appear as smoke or spirals or black walls. Often they will say that it is not like normal seeing, but when pressed cannot explain how it is different. This is not very useful for people trying to develop this ability in themselves. Unfortunately, many people who can 'see' energies in this way do not have the ability to recommend what needs to be done to rectify the problem. Some people who use kinesiology or dowsing find that they seem to develop the ability to 'see' these energies. It is likely that we all have this latent ability, but that it is more developed in some people than in others.

When I was very active in the geopathic stress field, I found that after a while I was able to sense these energies. It is inconvenient to be aware of these things when you are trying to go about your normal business, so I would 'switch off' this ability when it was not needed. On one occasion I had been in London for the weekend discussing geopathic energies with a group of like-minded people. I forgot to turn off this ability to see these energies once the discussions were over. An hour later I was driving home along the M5 motorway, when I suddenly saw a black wall in front of me. I slammed on the brakes, only to go through the 'wall' without anything untoward happening. It took me a few moments to realise that what I had 'seen' was almost certainly a geopathic phenomenon. I quickly turned off this awareness, and resolved to be more careful in future, as a major accident could so easily have happened.

Using A Map

Although those who sense energies usually need to go to the property, both dowsers and kinesiologists may prefer to look at a map or plan of a property rather than visit the property itself. Some practitioners like, where possible, to do both. A kinesiologist will usually use self-testing (see page 90), and a dowser will usually use a pendulum rather than the rods that are used for a site visit. Rolf Gordon (13) says he prefers to use a heavy pointed metal pendulum rather than a small crystal pendulum when map dowsing. Many of the kinesiologists who work solely from plans will generally still wish, if possible, to muscle test someone who lives or works at the site, or to have previously visited the site themselves.

Many clients prefer on-site analysis, because it seems to be more credible to them, but this may be practically difficult and expensive. There are also other drawbacks of on-site visits. Although it may result in a more accurate understanding of the energies involved, on-site exposure to the geopathic energies can lead to the practitioner becoming over-taxed and confused.

In the early day of undertaking geopathic stress consultations, I was acutely embarrassed about how disorientated I became as I walked through the area I had been asked to assess. Even in quite a small property I would lose all sense of where the front was. I learnt to tell clients about this problem before I entered the property. Otherwise their confidence faltered in this so-called expert who could not find her way back to the front entrance of the building. I also often developed pain in my lower back. Given Harvalik's work (page 87) this may have been my adrenal glands hurting rather than my back. Because of all this I came to prefer to do the analysis and recommendations using a map. In additional to a detailed plan of the property provided by the client, I also liked to look at a map of the area. This gave me both an intimate sense of the property itself and also a feeling for how it was located in its environment.

Maureen and Mike Rawles (31) always remotely map dowse a location prior to a visit, in order to have an 'overview of the earth energy', so helping them to prepare and understand the types of energies involved, particularly negative entity energy (page 51). This greatly reduces the probability of surprise, and minimises the time required on-site.

Visiting The Site

Some practitioners like to use a combination of plan analysis and site visits, whereas others will visit a site without looking at a plan first. Most practitioners will walk around the site in order to develop some sort of 'feel' for the place. The practitioner then starts to test the area, moving in a systematic way in order to cover the whole site. While doing this, they keep in mind all the different types of energy. As well as looking for negative energy lines, such as black lines, they also look for spirals and clouds. Not all geopathic phenomena are found at ground level. Energy drains, for example, can be located in mid-air. So this needs to be taken into account too. The findings are usually noted on a plan. Most practitioners develop different symbols for different types of energy. Particular attention is usually paid to the area directly below any beds or favourite chairs.   Working directly with geopathic energies in this way can be very draining, so many practitioners move away from the site they are examining for short rests, returning when they feel able.

Using Indices

Some practitioners like to work with a scale for geopathic stress. For instance, zero would indicate a complete absence of any form of geopathic stress and 100 would mean the area is geopathically saturated. The exact figure for the site is established using dowsing or kinesiology, and then the effect of any changes is monitored through the change in the index. Indices also allow the practitioner to track the effects of the geopathic stress on different people. (See page 78.) My book *Verbal Questioning Skills For Kinesiologists* covers more on this subject, and is a useful source of information and ideas both for kinesiologists and dowsers.

Accurate Results

Regardless of whether the practitioner is a dowser or kinesiologist, uses maps or undertakes site visits, it cannot be emphasised enough that both dowsing and kinesiology are 'operator sensitive', i.e. they are very dependent on the skills of the practitioner for the accuracy and validity of the results.

Some people feel that dowsing and kinesiology are more objective than the sensing the energies approach. This is not necessarily true: the dowsing rod and muscle testing are as open to influence, intentionally or unintentionally, as is the reaction of the person who sees energies.

Certainly the evidence from dowsing and kinesiology suggests that the person doing the dowsing or kinesiology is making the result happen. The pendulum, the rods and the subject's arm amplify small muscle changes. In the case of dowsing these muscle changes come from the arm of the person doing the testing. In the case of kinesiology it would appear that they could come from either the tester or the subject or both. When critics say that the person is moving the rods, the pendulum or the arm, this is probably true, but not in the sense that the sceptics mean. The critics usually mean that the practitioner is behaving dishonestly and performing some hoax. Reputable practitioners of dowsing and kinesiology strive to avoid influencing the results, so that the response is an amplification of unconscious changes in muscle response, rather than a conscious effort to make something happen.

Most practitioners act in good faith, but, unfortunately, some people influence the results they find. They usually do not do this intentionally. They subconsciously influence the results, because they believe strongly that they will find a particular type of energy at a particular site. The safeguards necessary to avoid this are primarily in the attitude of the practitioner. Of course, practitioners need to have some model or framework. They cannot just go into a house to find whatever is there, but it is important that the model is open to change and refutation. The practitioner needs to be skilful and open-minded. This is, quite a difficult combination of skills, but is surely akin to the attitude of mind that is espoused by the good researcher in any discipline: a desire for the findings to speak for themselves, rather than a determination to prove a particular pet theory or conclusion.

Coupled with this willingness to find what is there, it is important that the person doing the testing has a clear understanding of what they are looking for. Some years ago a client told me that there were reputed to be gold sovereigns in her house, hidden there by a long-dead sea captain. She asked if I could help her find them. I was reluctant to do this as I had no experience of locating objects in this way, but she persisted. In the end I agreed to do it as a light-hearted experiment. Using kinesiology I asked: 'Is there any hidden treasure in this house?' The response was positive, and so amid great excitement we tested to find the exact spot. Finally we came to the conclusion that the treasure was under a large chest freezer in the basement. When the chest freezer was removed, hidden treasure was indeed found: a one-pound coin that had obviously rolled under there at some point. She dug down into the earthen floor at a later date but found nothing further. My question had been about hidden treasure not about gold sovereigns. This story highlights how important it is to be clear about what you are asking. I should have asked the question: 'Are there any gold sovereigns buried in this house?' Testing for negative earth energies or geopathic energies without having a clear idea of what these are, is likely to lead to strange and garbled answers and confusion.

It is important that all the different types of geopathic energies are considered when checking an area for these energies. It has been found that when testing for geopathic energies it is usually not sufficient to have only a general concept of negative energy. At first sight, it would seem enough to hold in mind the concept of detrimental earth energies while testing. In practice this is often not satisfactory. There are many different energies within the universe, and a skilled dowser or kinesiologist can undoubtedly find many of these. In order to find the geopathic ones it is necessary to have a clear definition and 'feel' for what is involved, otherwise there is the risk of being overwhelmed and distracted by all the other energies occupying the same space. The practitioner's understanding of these energies influences what is found: the clearer and more comprehensive the understanding, the more accurate the testing.

People often feel that dowsing and kinesiology involve special 'gifts'. This is not true. Anyone who is willing to put in the time and effort can be taught to become competent in these techniques.

Undoubtedly though, as with any other skill, some people have more of an aptitude for it than others. Not all kinesiologists or dowsers have an interest in the problems of geopathic stress, so it is necessary to find out if a particular practitioner has an interest and experience in this field before engaging them.

CHAPTER 9

CORRECTING GEOPATHIC STRESS

Practitioners use many different ways to correct geopathic stress problems. Some of the differences reflect how different practitioners view these energies. Some practitioners believe that these energies are totally negative and need to be removed or neutralised in some way, whereas others seek to help the energies to flow in a less harmful way. Patrick MacManaway takes the second view. In his book *Dowsing For Health* he writes:

> Remember that the energy itself is neither good nor bad, and that something that may be harmful to us, can be helpful to other species.

Moving Beds

Correcting geopathic disturbances is not always difficult and complicated, although sometimes it can be. The first and simplest solution is always to move the bed or desk to another place. Sometimes people's health improves just from this one simple measure. Kathe Bachler's book *Earth Radiation* and Rolf Gordon's book *Are You Sleeping In A Safe Place?* describe many cases where doing only this has produced spectacular improvements in people's health and sense of well being. It is ironic that many sick people spend a lot of time in bed. If their illness is in part triggered by sleeping over geopathic energies, this will exacerbate their symptoms still further.

Practitioner Sylvia Bennett (05) helped a small boy with eczema.

She found through dowsing that he was sleeping over underground water. His bed was moved and the next day he woke up without itching. She needed to deal with some food problems for him too, but simply moving the bed produced an immediate improvement in his symptoms.

If simple measures like this do not work, it does not mean that geopathic stress is not a problem. It could be that the bed was moved from one harmful area to another. It could be that geopathic stress is a problem, but not in the bedroom area. Another possibility is that there are several geopathic areas in the house and simply moving the bed is not enough for the person to be aware of an improvement.

Unique Situations

Each site presents the practitioner with its own unique configuration of energies. Most practitioners recognise that each situation has to be treated as unique, depending on what is found during the analysis. There are many different types of geopathic energies, and there appears to be no one-to-one connection between which energies are found and how they are fixed. Each situation needs to be assessed individually. Most practitioners will assess the whole site, and then introduce solutions for the site as a whole rather than attempting to correct each energy individually.

Some practitioners, particularly manufacturers of proprietary devices, claim to be able to fix *all* geopathic energies. Most of these people are quite genuine when they say that they can do this, but I believe that with our limited understanding of these phenomena this claim should not be made.

An additional consideration is that some techniques that appear to correct geopathic stress may simply mask the problem, so that the negative energy cannot be detected, but is still harming the person. This is particularly dangerous because it lulls the person into a false belief that the building is now safe. Sometimes they initially respond, and then the old symptoms of ill health return. In this case it is likely that the initial response is a placebo reaction, but with time the harm from the geopathic energies becomes obvious again.

Individual Solutions

Some practitioners believe that the energy of the place can be corrected so that it will suit everyone, whereas others believe that a place has to be balanced for the specific people who live there. Roy and Ann Procter (30) take the second view:

> It's rather like different people needing different kinds of dwelling places at a physical level: one family would be best suited in a detached house in the country, another would feel more whole in an urban flat. So, we all need to live and work in an atmosphere which nourishes us at a subtler level.

My work with indices (see page 78) also suggests that it is necessary to consider the people who actually use the space that is being assessed.

Different Approaches

There are broadly five different approaches to fixing disturbed energies:

- Using artefacts (e.g. rods, stones, etc.)
- Using proprietary devices
- Using maps
- Using rituals and ceremonies
- Using the power of the practitioner's mind and intent

Some practitioners use a mixture of these, but many will use one particular type of intervention.

Using Artefacts

Geopathic energies can be handled in several different ways: they can be reflected or refracted, absorbed, blocked or transformed. Different types of geopathic energies need to be corrected in different ways. In one case reflecting an energy may be appropriate, whereas in another it may be appropriate to block it. It is vitally important, however, that whatever method is used, the undesirable energies are not changed in a way that is detrimental to others.

Different materials have different properties in relation to geopathic energies. Aluminium, graphite, quartz, elder and elm, for instance, can block the flow of energy when they are placed correctly. Lethbridge (see *The Essential T. C. Lethbridge*, edited by Graves and Hoult) called these 'energy interrupters'. Mirrors, when properly used, can reflect negative energies away from a building. These differences are not surprising when we consider how things have distinct properties in relation to electricity and magnetism. For example, water is a good conductor of electricity, whereas wood, rubber, glass and plastic are poor conductors. Similarly plastic, wood, glass, copper and aluminium cannot be magnetised, whereas iron and steel can be. If geopathic stress is, at least in part, an electromagnetic phenomenon, these properties of substances to become magnetised or to conduct electricity may well be relevant in choosing materials to counteract it.

The particular artefacts used for correcting geopathic stress are not necessarily placed directly over any negative energy line or spot. The exact positioning has to be established by careful testing using kinesiology or dowsing. Often several different objects will work in conjunction with each other, correcting the overall negative energy of the site.

Crystals, Wood & Other Artefacts

Crystals are probably used more frequently than any other artefacts. Crystals, particularly quartz, are seen as having special energy properties. In *Vibrational Medicine* Richard Gerber writes that quartz crystals will vibrate at different rates depending on what energy is put into the crystal. Pressure on the crystal will result in a different crystal vibration from when sound is beamed at it.

It is not totally clear how crystals bring about change, but one possibility is that the crystal is changing the frequency of the geopathic energies to one that is more acceptable to the humans exposed to it. It has also been suggested that crystals 'absorb' geopathic energies. Expensive beautiful crystals can be used, but, fortunately, this is not necessary. Crushed marble, which can be bought from some garden centres or from a monument maker, will do the job perfectly well at a fraction of the cost. As well as establishing exact location(s), the practitioner will also test for the type and amount of crystal to be used.

Most practitioners also give instructions for the crystals to be washed regularly to remove the accumulation of negative energy. The simplest way to do this is to place the crystal or crystals in a bucket and run water over them for about half an hour. How frequently this should be done, and the exact length of time for the cleaning process can be established by kinesiology or dowsing.

An engineer attended a workshop I taught on geopathic stress. He subsequently checked a riding stable for GS. The owner was particularly concerned because one of the horses was unpredictable and vicious. This was a riding school with a large clientele of small children, and the owner was considering having the horse put down. The engineer checked the stables and advised that two piles of crystals (4.5 kg / 10 lb in all) should be put in the stables at strategic spots. The owner was delighted to find that the horse's temper improved to such an extent that she was able to abandon any thought of putting the horse down. She also found that other horses had been affected. One mare, which had been particularly difficult to get into her box, now went in without any problem. Previously it had often taken up to half an hour. All the horses and ponies were generally less skittish in the yard once the GS had been corrected.

Mike and Maureen Rawles (31) feel that using large piles of crystals is unnecessary and is not working with the earth's energy. They use small crystals and pieces of wood placed in precise places on the edge of particular water or ley lines. They feel this still allows the energy lines to flow, but counteracts their detrimental effects.

David Cowan in his book *Safe As Houses* describes how he uses quartz crystals:

> If there is only a simple grid pattern of unhealthy waves present, with intersections in a bed for instance — if it is not practicable to move the bed to a safer place — then quartz crystals can be put down on the incoming waves to change them from unhealthy to healthy. Since unhealthy waves will not pass ... through windows, but instead enter indirectly, at the side of the glass, these are the best locations to place crystals. If you have a cluster or geode of crystals, such as amethyst or clear quartz, place one on the window ledge where you find the incoming wave. This can be done on any floor of a house or building, and will effectively clear both upper and lower storeys as well. Do this wherever you find the unhealthy waves entering key points in the house, where you sleep, sit, or stay for extended periods. Remember that window frames often have vertical wooden or metal parts where unhealthy waves will easily penetrate.

Tracy Longdon (26) uses various artefacts (as well as meditation) to correct geopathic energies:

I dowse to find out what the earth needs to heal it. I have a selection of 'pins' (twigs from trees), which I gained through a process of ceremony. I start with these, asking the 'do you want this one' question in my head for each pin, to establish which pin it wants. I then go through other items which represent the different elements, again asking 'do you want this' question for each set of items. If there is more than one choice for each type of item, I narrow it down with the same question. I use crystals for earth, a candle in a lamp for fire, salt for purification, a metal rod for metal and water for water. Sometimes the earth needs something from the actual house rather than from my kitbag. I position the items wanted on top of and around the healing point and then ask if it needs anything else. Normally it says 'yes', and I then ask if it needs some meditation, and it again normally says yes. I then sit and imagine the harmful earth energies being released through the pin. I can normally see a kind of 'mirage' effect at the top of the pin at this point. After about 5 minutes of meditation on this I check to find out if that's enough. When it is, I then check how long it needs to clear the geopathic stress and leave it for this amount of time.

Tracy gave me this example of her work:

Viv and her housemate went to a Vega therapist, and both were told that they were geopathically stressed. They were also told that the lines were in a 'Hartmann grid' configuration so that two lines were crossing under each of their beds. This meant that they could not move the beds away from the influence of the lines. Rather than move house they consulted me. I went to the house and used 'earth acupuncture' to remove the lines. Straight away they slept more soundly and felt they had more energy. Both of them went back to the Vega tester who confirmed they were no longer geopathically stressed.

The interesting thing about this case study was that about a month after I did it, a huge explosion happened (the largest in Europe) of a petroleum storage facility, which was very close to them. The explosion woke them both and actually moved the house. After that, one of the occupants stopped sleeping again. She went back to the Vega tester who said the geopathic stress had returned. She called me, and I dowsed remotely. I found that a line had in fact returned but was affecting only one of the beds. I remotely healed this from the plan without needing to return to the house and all was well afterwards. This was again confirmed by the Vega tester.

Mirrors

It is thought that a mirror can reflect a negative ray back onto itself, thereby cancelling out the charge on it. The exact size and placing of the mirror is important in order to achieve this. Most people, of course, have mirrors in their houses for reasons other than that of correcting geopathic stress. All mirrors can have an effect on geopathic energies, depending on their placing, so it may be necessary to take down a mirror or move it to another place as part of the correction process.

My easiest geopathic case of all was a simple matter of moving a mirror. The client had been experiencing stomach problems for some time. Initially I did not suspect geopathic stress, as we had previously checked her house and corrected the existing problems. Eventually, after drawing a blank over other possibilities, I decided to check the house again. Using kinesiology I checked and found that something had changed since the original analysis. When I looked at a plan of the house, I found a mirror was needed in the client's bedroom. My client looked surprised and then told me that there was a wardrobe on that wall. One of its sliding doors was mirrored. By sliding the doors the other way the mirror was then in the correct place to neutralise the geopathic energy. She then realised that when I had checked her house before, the wardrobe doors were in this beneficial position. Some months previously she had changed them over and that had coincided with the onset of her stomach symptoms. She went home, changed the doors back to the earlier position, and her stomach problems disappeared. The client was amazed and thrilled at this simple solution to her problems.

Aluminium Foil

Practitioners sometimes use aluminium foil. Normal aluminium foil bought for cooking may be adequate, providing several layers are used for robustness and any joins are overlapped. The foil must be checked regularly and any holes patched or the foil replaced.

One of my clients, a boy of 12, had problems with allergies. He was prone to headaches and recurring earache. He was also allergic to swimming pool water. On testing him I found that his lymph system needed strengthening, which I did using health kinesiology techniques. Initially we saw some improvement in his health, but, when this did not continue, I began to suspect geopathic problems. Testing confirmed this. Further testing indicated that the solution was to fasten a piece of aluminium foil approximately 1 metre by 1 metre (approximately 39 inches by 39 inches) at a carefully tested place on one inside wall of the house. The parents were, not surprisingly, sceptical that this could possibly have any effect, but were willing to do it and see what happened. They were delighted when their son's health problems disappeared.

Occasionally it is possible for either foil or a mirror to be used, but sometimes it has to be one or the other. Usually it is not necessary for either the foil or mirrors to be exposed. They can, if convenient, be hidden by furniture. Both can also usually be covered with wallpaper or paint without this affecting their function.

Plastic Sheeting

Rolf Gordon (13) suggests using thick plastic sheet or several layers of thin plastic sheeting (e.g. refuse bags) between the bed base and the mattress. He says that, though this will give immediate protection, the sheeting will need replacing every 1-2 weeks. Cork floor tiles are another alternative he suggests, but again these need replacing frequently.

Rods In The Ground

Sometimes rods are hammered into the ground at precise spots. The rods are usually made from solid copper or iron, with a diameter of at least 1.25 cms (0.5 inches). Rolf Gordon (13) recommends that the rods are about 35 cms (14 inches) long, but I found that the correct length varies from property to property, and so I always tested (using kinesiology) for the exact length. Often the rods have to be hammered in so that they are about 15 centimetres (approximately six inches) below the level of the ground. In one case it became evident that it was important to keep the space between the top of the rod and ground level clear, otherwise the benefit of the rods was severely diminished. Often there is a series of rods along one side of the house; all placed an equal distance apart.

One of my clients had to put a series of rods of a specific length into the ground, 0.3 metres (approximately 12 inches) away from an outer wall of the house. The owners of the house were amazed that the rods went into the ground just the right amount before a change in rock strata was encountered. Because of its hardness, this would have made further penetration difficult. Presumably the rods had to be this specific length to counteract the change in geology, which none of us knew about beforehand.

Mike and Maureen Rawles (31) do not use rods. They feel that this blocks the earth's energy rather than helping it to flow positively.

Colour

Colour can be used in many ways. Sometimes a wall needs painting a particular colour or a coloured light bulb needs to be placed in a particular place. The colour of light is related to the wavelength of the light waves. For instance, red has a longer wavelength than violet. Because of this different colours have different energy properties. These properties can be used to alter geopathic energies. The precise colour and location has to be determined by testing. Sometimes colour in the form of paint is appropriate and sometimes it has to be a coloured light.

Magnets

Some practitioners use magnets. They are usually 800 to 1200 gauss in strength, and magnetised in such a way that there is only one pole on each face of the magnet. Many magnets are magnetised through the ends. The magnetic strips used on doors are magnetised across the width but with alternating poles. Neither of these types of magnets will do. Specialist magnet companies provide suitable magnets. Magnets can be placed on walls, ceilings or floors to counteract geopathic problems. They are also used to counteract electromagnetic problems (see appendix 1).

Geometric Shapes & Models

Some practitioners use shapes. Pyramids are often chosen, but great care has to be taken as pyramids can amplify energy, and this applies whether the energy is positive or negative. Amplifying already detrimental energies is avoided by the practitioner testing carefully for the exact location in which to place the pyramid. Shapes can be made from many different materials, and the practitioner will usually test which ones are appropriate for a specific site.

Photographs

Occasionally a practitioner uses a photograph of the building. This could be a full colour photograph, a black and white photo or even a negative. This may have to be taken from a specific position. The photograph may need to be buried or put inside the house in a specific position. Often photographs appear to be used to cancel out the negative energies, but can be used for other reasons. Giulia Boden (06) described how she used a photograph for one property:

> A house that had been converted into a row of cottages, tested that that particular cottage needed a photo of the entire house in it – perhaps to feel whole?

Symbols

Many practitioners use symbols to alter the feel and quality of both negative and positive energy. Careful testing through dowsing or kinesiology can determine the size, background colour and so on. Some practitioners will devise symbols themselves, whereas others will use pre-existing symbols.

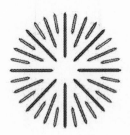 I often used a set of 12 symbols designed by Heather Willings (27), called *Health Through The Eyes*. Each of these symbols on a card strengthens a particular acupuncture meridian. Heather found the twelve symbols through a combination of dowsing, intuition and meditation. If a person has an imbalance in a particular

meridian, looking at the relevant symbol for a little while will re-balance the meridian. People are often attracted to the symbol that they need to re-balance their energy system. The symbol named 'Starburst' (see below) can correct imbalances in the stomach meridian and 'Arrowheads' supports the kidney meridian. Each card is also related to particular emotional qualities. 'Starburst' is used for confidence, perseverance, acceptance of what is necessary and the assurance to overcome adversity. It can also help free blocked energy and cleanse negative emotions. 'Arrowheads' helps engender decisiveness, tenacity, willpower and strength to assume responsibility. It is also said to harmonise physical and spiritual energy.

I found that these cards were also useful for correcting geopathic energies, testing to find the correct one or ones, and exactly where in the property they needed to be placed. When I am travelling, I usually carry a pack of these cards with me. They can be very useful for temporarily correcting geopathic energies in rooms I sleep in on my travels. Some practitioners who work to change geopathic stress using their mind or intent also use symbols, but these are usually imagined rather than actual symbols. (See page 118.)

Different practitioners have a fondness for particular artefacts, but these are some of the most commonly used ones.

Using Essences

Some practitioners use essences, such as the Bach flower remedies, to spray in an affected area. This may be particularly effective where the paranormal and/or trapped emotions are involved. The practitioner may chose one or more essences according to the 'mood' of the place, or may use one specifically designed for that purpose, e.g. Space Clearing Mist from Australian Bush Essences (04).

Alaskan Flower Essences (01) have a group of sprays called Sacred Space Sprays that are a blend of flower, gem, and environmental essences. The one called Guardian may be particularly useful:

> Guardian sets a grounded and radiant energy into the space that helps each person who enters move into their center and maintain a connection to the source of their protection, their own inner light.

On their web site they suggest a complete ritual for using this and other essences to clear and protect spaces.

Chris Tivey of Creative Building Solutions (10) uses blended gem and flower essences:

> I use essences not only for clearing areas affected by the geopsychic realms [paranormal], but also for electromagnetic radiation, environmental pollution and geopathic stress. I choose the appropriate remedies by pendulum dowsing and tend to use a range produced by Josephine Harris of Central Life Harmony [09]. Space Clear 1 (Geopathic) for example contains essences of amethyst, Herkimer diamond, diamond, brown jasper and aragonite, and has been found to be effective in blocking and alleviating geopathic stress. It also stabilises and heals the earth chakra and environment. The vibration of the crystalline structure of the gems is retained within the essences that harmonise the specific energies of the environmentally stressed area. I also recommend protective aura sprays for areas such as work places, schools and hospitals where it may be difficult to carry out remedial work.

Proprietary Devices

There are various devices sold by different companies specifically to correct geopathic stress. Sceptics usually say these work as a placebo, but almost all of them are very unimpressive when first seen. They do not immediately instil confidence. Sometimes the accompanying literature is far from glossy. If I were setting out to design an effective placebo, I would not do it like this.

It is impossible to cover all the devices that are currently available, so this section can only give a flavour of what may be useful.

Geomack

Geomack (15) sell several different products to:

> to create a protective shield of energy that keeps external radiation at bay while filling the place with human friendly frequencies.

The portable Energia 601, cover a diameter of 3 metres (10 feet) around the unit, and the E9001 Pure covers up to 200 sq metres (2000 square feet). The company has designed all the units to protect against both geopathic stress and electromagnetic pollution. They also have an EP 1400, which is designed to work in areas were there are extremely high levels of electromagnetic pollution (see appendix 1) from the close proximity of mobile phone masts, electric pylons, etc. They offer a five-month money back guarantee on all their units, but say that less than 1% are returned.

Gabrielle Harvey-Jones, the wife of a former chairman of the large UK company ICI, installed two units in their barn conversion at the suggestion of a friend. 4 years later she wrote a letter to Geomack:

> We are delighted with them and the effect they have had on many aspects of our daily lives. I have two long standing physical conditions, Late Effect Polio and Multiple Sclerosis, and I noticed improvements in both conditions within a week. We both find that we sleep much better, and the whole atmosphere of the house is so peaceful that all our friends remark on it.

The live blood analysis (see page 6) also offers an interesting confirmation of the effectiveness of this device.

GFD-1 & 2

The GFD-1 and 2 (also called SFT Field Resonators) are devices from Subtle Field Technologies (34). The units are designed to

produce a holograph field that protects the human bio-magnetic system from negative electro-magnetic fields, and microwave electro-magnetic radiation.

The GFD-1 covers an area of 500 square metres and the GFD-2 covers 800 square metres. Gary Johnson of Subtle Field Technologies told me about how he helped a client by using rods and one of these devices:

Mrs R. from Bow, London contacted me regarding problems in her house, especially, the kitchen. She had been very unwell for several years with M.E type symptoms. Also her husband suffered from restless painful legs when he sat for too long in a particular chair in their lounge. I was called out to test for any negative energy problems in the house. The house was checked by using dowsing and divining rods, and two geopathic stress lines were found.

Both of the geopathic stress lines were caused by geological faults (earth movement). One of the fault lines ran the length of the house and half the width. The second fault line ran at 85 degrees across the first. Where the two fault lines crossed (in the kitchen) is where Mrs R. always complained of a 'numb cold feeling'

Two courses of action were necessary to neutralise the negative effects of geopathic stress at this house. Initially 1 and 1.5 metre iron and brass rods were sunk into the ground at certain positions in the front and rear gardens. This action neutralised the geopathic radiation in both geological lines, but where the two lines crossed was still causing the numb cold feelings in Mrs R. A SFT-4 protection device was placed in the kitchen area, which finally resolved the case. Mrs R's numb cold feeling disappeared and her husband's legs improved.

Helios Device

These are sold by Healthy Home (23). Gina Lazenby, writer and owner of Healthy Home, describes them:

> You simply plug this into an electrical socket to change the frequencies of your home to resonate with the beneficial wavelengths of the earth. You won't feel anything but immediately you will start to sleep deeper and wake up feeling more refreshed and full of vitality. Your immune system will no longer be suppressed and this will help to improve your condition if you are ill.

Christine Houghton, a therapist, is very impressed with the device:

> I live in a 150-year-old house where streams run under the property and it was once a mining community. Geopathic stress is a big issue in this area, I have always been concerned about the environment in which I live so from the moment I experienced the Helios Home Harmoniser machine at a demonstration I knew it was what my house needed. How right I was, almost from the first moment the Helios was plugged in I felt the difference. My husband now sleeps the whole night through whereas before he was having difficulty sleeping and the side effect of this is that his energy levels have risen dramatically. For me the Helios is one of the most amazing machines on the market, every home should have one. Recently, my friend said she was having problems so I lent the machine to her. Amazingly, within just a few days, at least half a dozen friends told her that her home felt different.

Neutralec Neutraliser

The origin of this device from Neuralec Limited (28) is very interesting. Ian Hardiman was a carpet consultant undertaking independent carpet inspections for carpet manufacturers. He would go to the houses of the carpet customers to assess the validity of complaints. He found that one problem kept on occurring: the carpet would appear to have a blotchy watermark – an optical illusion caused by the pile being displaced. This could occur in areas where people were not walking. Even when the carpet was replaced, the problem would recur. Ian realised that the problem was caused by electrical appliances:

> Investigations in consumer and commercial premises soon enabled me to realise certain common factors involved in these "Phenomenon" Shading complaints. Often, I would see that shading occurred adjacent to radiators, Hi-Fi systems, battery chargers and even that an electrical or electronic appliance was in use, in a room above where a problem exists!

He teamed up with his brother Michael, who has a background in the nuclear industry, and developed a device to correct the problem. This was plugged into an electrical socket and used the mains earth as the transmission device. Once these were in use, people started to phone Ian to tell him how well they were feeling, and he realised that the neutraliser was achieving more than just counteracting a carpet problem. Now he sells more of the neutralisers to people concerned about their health than to people concerned about their carpets.

They have also developed a model that can be worn to protect against EMF fields. The neutraliser was not designed to counteract geopathic stress, but Ian told me he believes it is correcting both EMF and GS problems.

The RadiTech

The RadiTech is designed by Rolf Gordon of Dulwich Health (13). This unit is plugged into an electrical socket, but does not use any electricity. It uses the existing electrical wiring to 'neutralise' the geopathic stress in the building. It is designed to protect the building from geopathic stress and reduce problems with electromagnetic pollution (see appendix 1). There are different RadiTechs for different situations, including one for use in the car and one for large buildings and institutions. The makers say:

The RadiTech incorporates electronics, powerful magnets and cables in very accurately (sic) patterns embedded in special (sic) formulated mastic.

The RadiTech comes with a full money back guarantee. Rolf Gordon who designed the RadiTech told me:

We've sold tens of thousands and probably got 1% back.

The RadiTech only works while it is plugged in. I talked to a man whose wife had bought a RadiTech and believed it helped her sleep better. He was extremely sceptical about this and felt it was helping her because she believed it would. He decided to test this out. He unplugged the RadiTech without telling her, and she immediately started sleeping much worse again. He was very impressed by this and concluded that the RadiTech must be working in some way he did not understand.

The Dulwich Health literature includes many examples of the successful use of a RadiTech. For example:

A manager in charge of an upper floor in Centre Point, the tall London office building, confirmed his large sales staff had become more enthusiastic after a RadiTech was installed unknown to his staff.

Mrs. N Thompson, Kent "I was going to have an operation for an old back problem, but within three weeks of having the RadiTech I canceled (sic) the operation and went on a skiing holiday instead."

Red Nine Harmoniser

Applied Energetic Wisdom (03) produces a Red Nine harmoniser for homes and offices. Tony G. Mills describes it in this way:

It has 3 types of crystals with specific properties that are placed strategically on a geometrically charged grid. This combination allows the protective energy emitted by the harmoniser to cover approximately an area of 60 yards radius (sufficient for most homes and offices). It reduces aches and pains and emotional stress, incidences of headaches, cot deaths (SIDS) and chronic fatigue symptoms. Increases energy, better concentration, strengthens immune system and improves sleep patterns.

Tony sometimes uses a combination of energy work and the harmoniser:

> For a long period Janet's next-door neighbours would violently argue most nights of the week. Once Janet and her house were harmonised, the quarrelling stopped the next day.

Fixing Remotely Using Maps

Maps can be used as part of the analysis (see page 91), but some practitioners also use them as part of the correction process. Some practitioners place crystals, coins and other artefacts on a map of the site rather than at the actual site itself. This map may be kept by the practitioner or given to the client.

Some years ago I established through kinesiology that energy drains (see page 45) could also be cleared using numbers on a map. This may seem a little strange, but every number seems to have a vibrational rate that may correspond with some other phenomenon. I discovered that the number for a fully functioning drain, for example, is 2222222, and the rate to unblock a drain remotely is 311313. Using numbers to unblock drains needs to be done by an experienced practitioner, as the numbers need to be used in precise ways. Using them inappropriately can lead to the energies becoming even more disturbed.

Using Rituals And Ceremonies

Ceremonies are sometimes appropriate for correcting geopathic energies. Some religions have a history of using ceremonies in connection with the paranormal, but it is possible to use ceremonies without any religious connotations at all. Sadly, for some people the term 'ceremony' or' 'ritual' implies some association with devil worship. Used in the context of geopathic work, they have absolutely no involvement with black magic.

Practitioners may use pre-existing rituals. They may come from a mainstream religious source, or from Celtic, Native American or other shamanic practices. Some practitioners devise their own rituals, either by testing or intuitively. The ritual may include music, candles, essential oils, burning herbs, visualisation, dance and more.

Giulia Boden (06) gave me this interesting example of the use of ritual and ceremony:

> The house had been repossessed from the previous owners. It was in a very bad state of repair, and the new owners had found pornography in it. This plus a very GS'd house made for a major overhaul in all areas. I came across a ley line that turned out to be a funeral path running through the house. It was straight and then formed a rectangle and then continued on its way in the direction of the church. Reading up on this I found out that a funeral procession would often stop on the way to the church. The coffin would be put down while prayers were said over it. Alternatively people might walk around the coffin several times to ward off spirits. The rectangular 'kink' that I had found in the line represented this.
>
> I tested that the owner had to walk the pathway through her house on her own. She needed to do this solemnly with a candle and some incense. Then on May Day, which happened to be at this time, she and her whole family had to make wreaths of flowers, attach ribbons, and dance their way together along the path. A friend commented afterwards that she thought they had redecorated which they hadn't at that point, and she felt the energy had really lightened and shifted.
>
> I also did some distant healing work on the place, and the following day all the people they had been waiting for to plaster, plumb and transform the kitchen came.

In my experience blocked energy drains (see page 45) can usually be fixed using rituals. Kinesiology or dowsing is used to establish the exact detail of the ritual, but a common format seems to be a certain number of people (usually women), forming a circle by holding hands and walking a specific number of times around the energy drain. Sometimes the people involved have to visualise something at the same time (in one case a red poppy). Another alternative is using sound in some way. This ritual needs to be repeated on a regular basis.

Giulia Boden (06) describes how it feels when an energy drain is cleared:

> ... experiencing the surge in energy that occurs when you do this, like a mill wheel that has long been stuck and is then wound into motion feeling as though water were coursing through it!

This method of energy correction is particularly interesting in the light of Fidler's discussion of the dream he had of people dancing around a standing stone in order to charge it (*Ley Lines*). The fact that the sex of the participants is often important ties in with Lethbridge's work on energetically charging stones, where the sex of the charger is clearly transmitted to the stone (see *The Essential T. C. Lethbridge*, edited by Graves and Hoult).

Sometimes the problem with the drain is not the drain itself, but the fact that it has been switched off. Usually this involves moving household appliances inadvertently located over the switch associated with the drain. (See page 45).

Using The Power Of The Practitioner's Mind And Intent

This may be the method that the general public find hardest to accept, because it is arguably the most implausible. To the sceptic it can seem like someone creating something with their mind/imagination and then saying they have fixed this non-existent phenomenon with their mind. No wonder they are not impressed. However, a more detailed look at what is going on, can reward the inquirer with some intriguing insights.

There is an extremely interesting article in the *Journal Of Alternative And Complementary Medicine* (Vol 11, Number 5, 2005) with the title 'Spooky Action At A Distance: Physics, Psi & Distant Healing'. It was Einstein who first used the phrase 'spooky actions at a distance' to describe his unhappiness at some of the ideas of quantum mechanics. The article by Drew Leder starts by describing how 'spooky actions at a distance' – such as telepathy, telekinesis, clairvoyance, distant healing and prayer – have been documented and are now being studied by some scientists. The author says that there is a barrier to this work being taken seriously, because it is seen as being 'fundamentally incompatible with the scientific world view'. He goes on to suggest that this should not be the case and sets out four possible 'interpretative frameworks' in which these spooky actions at a distance could be incorporated into scientific understanding.

He looks at these four models (energetic transmission, path facilitation, nonlocal entanglement and actualization of potential), explaining the advantages and problems of each. Two of these models, path facilitation and actualization of potential, offer some insights into how the practitioner may be able to redirect and change geopathic energies, although the article itself is talking about the actions of healers.

Leder explains that gravitational pull is exerted by large objects such as the earth, and can be seen to be a 'spooky action at a distance'. He writes:

> Like a bowling ball lying on a mattress, a star or planet warps the universe around it and draws other objects towards it.

He discusses the possibility of powerful healers (or a group of people focussed on a similar outcome) having an effect akin to the gravitational pull of a very large object. The healer or group facilitate a path to a particular outcome. The analogy is not perfect. He points out that unlike the gravitational pull of the earth; for example, the powerful healer does not affect all who are within his/their range, but only the object of the activity. Nevertheless, this does give some insight into how GS practitioners might bend and distort energies.

The second of Leder's frameworks that may be relevant here is actualization of potential. In quantum mechanics the measurer is seen as influencing the outcome:

> the particle cannot be said to have a definite location before measurement.

The act of measuring gives the particle a definite attribute rather than a range of possibilities. The healer in this version is acting like the measurer. Leder uses the example of someone with a cancer that typically has a survival rate of 20%:

> This is analogous to a particle that has a 20% chance of being found here.

The healer through intention/prayer affects whether the event (death from cancer) will be found here (within this client). The healer's work has shifted the balance so that one outcome is more likely than another. Again this can be seen to parallel the work of geopathic specialists who claim to change energies with their mind or intent. They may make the outcome of no or few geopathic energies more probable by their intervention.

Many, but not all, of the practitioners who work with intent feel that they have some spirit guide, guru or some connection with divine energy in their work. Ann and Roy Procter (30) were trained initially to hammer lengths of heavy angle iron into the ground in a spot determined very precisely by dowsing, but over time they have changed to correcting geopathic energies through intent. In their book *Healing Sick Houses* they talk about the development of their work, and how, after a visit by Roy to Mother Meera, 'a special avatar person born in India and now living in Germany', they are finding it much easier to achieve results.

Many practitioners are unwilling or unable to explain exactly how they use their intent to fix geopathic stress problems, but David Furlong in his book *Earth Energies* summarises the process he uses in the following way:

> To correct any imbalances use a *Celtic Cross* for any problems that stem from within the Earth; use a *golden pyramid* for those problems that flow above the Earth. In all cases communicate with the elemental forces of the area and get their help whenever you can.

******

Regardless of what assessment and remedial action is taken, it is important to monitor the situation from time to time. Geopathic stress can change with time for reasons that are not really understood, although seasonal factors certainly play a part. In Canada, for example, Jimmy Scott (16) has found that there can be significant differences in geopathic energies between winter and summer in areas where the ground freezes to a considerable depth in the winter.

There are other reasons for changing or fluctuating geopathic situations. Alterations or redecoration within a house can change the existing situation by, for instance, deflecting or concentrating these harmful energies in different areas within the house. Work in nearby buildings may also cause problems in the same way. For all these reasons it is important to monitor what is happening and to carry out further remedial work whenever necessary.

Mike Rawles of Dragonstone (31) told me this interesting story about how quickly things can change. It was almost as if this happened because the very sceptical client needed personal evidence of the reality of geopathic stress.

> The occupants of the house had been told that the house had both geopathic stress issues (by a kinesiologist) and ghostly history (from local informants). The owners were typically sceptical of both scenarios, but were concerned enough to ask Dragonstone to look into the issue. The house was first remotely map dowsed , in order to identify the types of earth energy involved, and to provide a report of our considered opinion .... this resulted in an on-site visit to balance the house's negative energies. This visit entailed converting the negative earth energies to white light, space clearing the associated negative energy hosted by the house [see page 51], and making safe the edges of the white light yin energy lines. After approximately six hours on-site we departed back home. The following morning we had an urgent telephone call: neither she nor her daughter had slept that night. A quick remote dowsing investigation showed that a white light energy line (yang ley-type line) had evolved since the energies were changed, causing the sleep disturbance. This resulted in an immediate return, to make safe the line's edge, convincing a once unsure client, that there is definitely something very significant in the influences of earth energy upon our lives and health.

Fortunately most sites do not need further remedial work as quickly as this, but nevertheless it is important to monitor the situation. Dragonstone, for example, recommend a three-monthly check up process to make sure all is still well.

CHAPTER 10

SELF HELP & PROTECTION FOR THE INDIVIDUAL

Helping People To Be Less Susceptible To Geopathic Energies

Geopathic stress practitioners often concentrate on reducing or eliminating the geopathic energies within a property, but it is important, where possible, to help people to cope better with any geopathic energies that they encounter. People are exposed to geopathic energies as they go about their normal lives even if their home is clear.

Unfortunately one of the problems of being consistently exposed to geopathic stress is that it often seems to undermine a sufferer's ability to make and carry out decisions. In consequence of this many people will need help in doing whatever is necessary to correct their home or work place. They can find even the most simple of self-help measures difficult to carry out. They frequently seem to lack the necessary energy and determination to change things so that they are no longer disturbed by these energies.

The best way I know of making people permanently more robust to geopathic energies is using techniques from health kinesiology (HK). Health kinesiologists (16 and 17) use the term energy control system to refer to the part of the energy system that is often affected by geopathic energies. This is part of the central control process for subtle energy within the body, and so is of fundamental importance. HK has a range of correcting procedures that rebalance the energy control system, making it more robust and capable of withstanding geopathic energies. Before I was introduced to HK in 1987 I was very susceptible to geopathic disturbances, but through working in this area my health and robustness has increased immeasurably. My book on health kinesiology has a lot more information on this treatment system.

Other therapies can be used to help clients suffering from GS problems. Sylvie Lenoir (24) worked with a dowser to both help the client and fix the environment:

> Isabel came to my practice for the first time on February the 11th 2005. She had been experiencing sleeping difficulties since she was born. Isabel is now 10 years old. She looked very old. The areas under her eyes were very dark. Her mother, Mande, told me that Isabel could only sleep under histamine tablets and for 2 hours only in 24 hours. The lack of sleep aggravated her eczema and asthma. The parents tried everything with doctors and with other alternative therapies without success. They came to my practice, very sceptical about the help I could bring. Since Isabel's birth, the parents have been living in the same house and Isabel always in the same bedroom. Only the bed changed place.
>
> Isabel had stopped growing and putting on weight. She was two years behind at school because she was so exhausted all the time, she could not learn or understand a lot. She could read but did not understand what she was reading. The parents were very concerned for her future. Doing her homework always triggered arguments and required a lot of effort.
>
> At this first visit, I dowsed to know what was the cause of her inability to sleep. I found out that she was suffering from geopathic stress. Isabel was sleeping on a negative ley-line, which was affecting her endocrine system and the pineal gland in particular. Her parasympathetic system was not working very well either. The geopathic stress was also cutting-off most of the essential fatty acids,

hormones, tissue salts, minerals and vitamins required for the proper function of the body.

Once I found the cause of her problem, I selected some remedies that could lift that cause. I made homeopathic tablets of those remedies, which I tapped on very precise points on her body. The night after my treatment, she slept properly for the first time since she was born.

I also suggested the parents to phone a professional dowser who could deal with the energies of their house. The report from the professional dowser said that "he found a wide energy line, parallel with the road, about 12 feet wide, running through the front garden and through the front wall of the house. The line edge was about 7 feet into the sitting room and covered Isabel's bed. Muscle testing revealed that the mother and Isabel were adversely affected by this line (the father was not present at the time of the muscle tests). In Isabel's room was a TV and video, an electric organ and worst of all, a SKY TV dish about 3 feet from Isabel's head on the outside wall." The dowser suggested all electrical equipment to be unplugged at night or when not in use and the TV dish moved. The bed was moved to another position too. He changed the frequency of the energy line so that it would benefit Isabel's health.

Isabel has never had sleeping problems since that day. Now that her body can properly perform its healing and repairing activities at night, she has started to grow again and put on weight. She has caught up at school with the other pupils.

Overall Health And Geopathic Stress

As well as seeking help from a suitably qualified practitioner, individuals can do much to help themselves. An individual's general health will affect their ability to resist the effects of geopathic stress. The healthier we are the less susceptible we are to all sorts of geopathic energies. This, of course, applies to any form of stress or toxic overload in our lives. Many people are looking for a single cause for an illness, but, in general, things are much less simple. For most diseases a number of different factors come together to bring about imbalance. It is not possible to say that one factor is the *cause* of the disease. It is the sum total of these which pushes a person over the threshold into illness and symptoms of disease.

Although this book, by its nature, is focusing on geopathic stress, it is important to realise that this is just one of several factors which contribute to a given person's ill health. I am not in any way suggesting that geopathic stress is THE cause of illnesses, but rather it should be seen as a major contributing factor in many health problems. The role of these factors in ill health can be seen like a bucket, (diagram) which fills with a certain amount of water every time one of these factors is present. So, if there is severe and long-lasting geopathic stress, a lot of water goes in the bucket. If more limited exposure happens, a small amount goes into the bucket. Similarly for all the other factors. Symptoms occur when the bucket overflows. It can seem that whatever caused the bucket to overflow is the cause of the symptoms or illness, but this is not necessarily so. All the different factors that filled the bucket may need to be considered in order to return the person to full health.

Geopathic stress should be seen as being part of the load on an individual. Other factors, such as environmental pollution (from car exhaust, tobacco smoke and other air borne substances), chemicals in food and water, allergies, a poor diet, lack of exercise, exposure to viruses and bacteria, electromagnetic pollution (appendix 1), emotional and financial problems and many other factors combine to undermine an individual's health. Intervention in any of these areas can lead to an improvement in health and help reduce the person's sensitivity to geopathic stress. When the body is being affected by many different stresses, it can be likened to an army having to fight on many different fronts.

Even if the house and workspace are corrected some sick people still do not regain their former good health. This may be because the geopathic stress has so undermined their body's functioning that treatment needs to be undertaken to strengthen the body and re-balance it. It is similar to a situation where a fuse blows in an electricity circuit because one too many appliances are plugged into the circuit. Removing the final appliance which caused the fuse to blow is not sufficient to get the system working again: one or more fuses also have to be replaced. To return to our bucket analogy, it is not sufficient just to stop putting more water in the bucket. The bucket has to be emptied. This can be done by consulting a reputable health practitioner, who will work to correct the destruction caused by exposure to the geopathic stress.

Free Radicals And Antioxidants

One very important general health measure is to ensure an adequate intake of antioxidants to protect the body against free radical activity. Free radical activity is seen as being at least partly responsible for the ageing process. It is implicated in degenerative arthritis, cardiovascular disease and cancer.

Free radicals are produced normally as a by-product of the body metabolising oxygen and other chemicals. Smoking, sunbathing, eating a lot of fried food, infections, excessive exercise, stress, radiation and polluted environments can all cause an excess of free radicals. Professor Gerald Scott of Aston University specialises in the understanding of free radicals. He told a public enquiry in Yorkshire that power line EMFs increase free radical activity within the body. It may also be that geopathic stress encourages free radical production.

Free radical molecules are highly unstable and seek to combine with other molecules in the body in a destructive manner. The process is similar to what happens when a cut apple becomes brown if left exposed to the air. Antioxidants bind with the free radicals, so stopping the free radicals attacking cell membranes and tissue linings. For this reason antioxidants are often known as free radical scavengers.

Vitamins A (in the form of beta-carotene), vitamins C and E, the mineral selenium, enzymes such as superoxide dismutase and the amino acid glutathione act as antioxidants. Fruit and vegetables contain antioxidants such as lycopene, so it is important to include plenty of these in the diet. Current government campaigns to encourage people to eat a lot more fruit and vegetables are in part because they contain antioxidants. There are also now many antioxidant supplement formulas on the market offering combinations of these different nutrients in a single tablet.

Reducing Exposure To Electromagnetic Pollution

It is advisable to reduce the amount of exposure to electromagnetic pollution particularly while sleeping. This will reduce the overload on the body, and make it easier to fight geopathic stress. (See appendix 1)

Essences

Essences can be sprayed in a building, and many can also be taken to help people to be less sensitive to geopathic stress. Alaskan Essences Guardian (see page 110), for example, can be used in both ways.

Devices For Individual Protection Against GS

There are many devices now being sold offering protection against geopathic stress and/or electromagnetic pollution. Most appear to offer some protection against some forms of geopathic stress, but it is doubtful if any of them protect against *all* forms of it. This does not mean that they are not useful things to have, but it is important that having one does not lull the owner into a false sense of security that they are totally protected. Owning one of these is not a substitute for putting the house or work place right. Many suppliers will offer a money-back guarantee, allowing the device to be tested with the minimum financial risk to the purchaser.

Even if the home and work place were corrected, wearing one of these devices would be an excellent idea for anyone who is particularly susceptible to GS. These devices are also useful if it is not possible to correct the geopathic problem for some reason, as can happen in some work situations.

Life Transformers

One such device is a geopathic stress Life Transformer (16 and 39). These were developed by Dr Jimmy Scott (16), the originator of health kinesiology. He has developed a whole series of Life Transformers to help people with a wide variety of problems, e.g. overcoming fears, smoothing the emotions, improving the memory, and so on. Each Life Transformer is a crystal that has been specifically programmed to help the wearer deal with a particular problem. Each programmed crystal emits specific energy patterns. Dr Scott found that rose quartz was the best crystal to hold the programme for the geopathic stress Life Transformer. The crystal is generally worn over the upper breastbone. While not protecting against all forms of GS, the geopathic stress Life Transformer does give some real protection against various types of negative energy.

Geomack

This company produce a portable Energia 601, which covers a

diameter of 1.5 metres (5 feet) around the unit. This can be carried in a briefcase or bag and placed on the floor or on a table whenever needed.

Pulsors

These were developed by Dr George Yeo in the 1960's. They are made from purified 'microcrystals' and are designed 'to resonate with the subtle energy vibrations that affect our sense of well-being'. There are various pulsors designed for particular situations including negative environmental energies, healing and aura protection. In the UK these are sold by the Wholistic Research Company (39).

Degaussing The Body

One treatment that seems to work well for many people is to degauss the body. The gauss is a unit for measuring the strength of a magnetic field. Degaussing means to demagnetise. In individuals who are particularly sensitive to geopathic stress and electromagnetic fields, degaussing the body can be helpful. It is also helpful for the many people who are prone to static electric shocks, or who are 'addicted' to television and/or video games. Dr Jimmy Scott (16) developed this technique as part of health kinesiology. It does not correct the geopathic problem, but allows most people to function better in a geopathically stressed environment.

It can be simply done using an alternating electric motor. Probably the most convenient device to use is a hair drier. The hair drier is switched on. The exact setting is irrelevant. The hair drier is then run over the whole body with the barrel of the hair drier against the body. This usually needs to be done on a regular basis. Small babies are sometimes frightened if you attempt to do this to them, so in this case it may be better to purchase a tape head demagnetiser, as these are totally silent in use. These are normally used to de-magnetise recording equipment, It is now possible to purchase cassettes to demagnetise tape recorders. These are *not* suitable. It is the more old-fashioned unit that plugs into an electric socket that is required. It is important that people should not be carrying credit cards or other cards with magnetic strips while this procedure is carried out. The degaussing is likely to affect the magnetic strip and make the card useless. Susceptible people may need to degauss about once a week.

GS Addiction

Some people appear to become addicted to geopathic stress, or at least to a certain level of GS. Often their favourite chair will be over the worst point in the house. If they move house, they may choose one with virtually identical problems. With these people their symptoms have not got worse or suddenly appeared since moving to their present home; they were also exposed to the same factors before, and, in all probability, their health has continually declined.

When the geopathic stress is corrected these people may exhibit a temporary worsening of their symptoms or even different symptoms. This usually only lasts for a few days. This is similar to what happens when someone gives up cigarettes – the person feels worse before they feel better.

At first sight this seems a peculiar phenomenon that we should 'like' things that are bad for us. However, you only have to think about cigarette smoking and drug abuse to know that this can occur. There are physiological reasons for this. Endorphins are the body's painkillers; our natural, biological equivalent to morphine. Geopathic stress may increase the body's production of endorphins. Unfortunately endorphins are addictive if produced over a long enough period of time. Just such a situation may exist when an individual works or lives in an area of high geopathic stress. So if the situation is corrected, and endorphin production is reduced suddenly, the person may exhibit symptoms of feeling worse. They are going through a process equivalent to that of drug withdrawal. This is not a good reason for not fixing GS problems, because in the long run the person is likely to feel much worse if it is not fixed. The reaction to the change in endorphin levels is temporary in nature.

Rolf Gordon (13) offers a different explanation of why some people feel worse when the geopathic problem is first corrected. He believes that toxins are being released from the body, and that this usually disappears within the first week.

If the people in the building continue to feel worse, this suggests that the manner of fixing the GS may not have been correct in its entirety, and that some adjustments are necessary. This may mean doing additional things to the house or relocating some of the corrective devices.

CHAPTER 11

CONCLUSIONS

Inevitably some of what has been written in this book is speculative in nature. There is not enough evidence yet to convince sceptics. Unfortunately many of the people working most successfully in this area are extremely modest and do not publish (or even publicise) their results. Yet it is vital that this should be done, so that the evidence can mount.

The Legal Question

One interesting development may be in the legal arena. If the concept of geopathic stress and its negative impact on health becomes accepted, there will need to be legal test cases to establish who is responsible for correcting any GS problems. It may well be that responsibility for geopathic stress problems will have to be written into the lease in the same way that responsibility for the external maintenance of a building now is. Similarly in new housing developments it will need to be established if legally it is the builders' responsibility to check on any possible geopathic stress problems both before and while building houses.

The two case studies on pages 18 and 19 must give any employer food for thought. Sickness and absenteeism are a drain on a company's profitability. Good employers will also be concerned about the human cost of this. Employees already take employers to court over working conditions that impinge on their health.

One day an employee or group of employees may mount a test case, claiming that geopathic stress has damaged their health.

GS & The Sceptics

It is clear to me that if you asked ten different GS practitioners to assess the same property, you would be likely to get ten different analyses and ten different solutions. Surely this suggests that this is just a mental construct with no validity? Maybe to the cynic it also suggests that these people are charlatans, robbing the gullible of their money and spreading unfounded alarm. Yet if the evidence presented in this book is reviewed dispassionately, this conclusion is not so easily reached.

The predictive studies by myself (page 18) and Giulia Boden (page 19) in business settings, which identified accurately where sick people would be working are difficult to explain away. What about the challenge that I successfully met to predict where people with headaches would be sitting in a lecture theatre (page 5)? How could I have known that the man on the TV programme suffered with leg or back problems, and that someone in the house probably had migraines (page 78)? Can the sceptics explain why the local cats all stopped congregating in a garden (just as I predicted, see page 22) once the GS was fixed in the house? What do the cynics have to say about the engineer who dowsed a negative energy line in a park and then looked up and saw all the trees as far as the horizon bending away from it? (See page 24.) What about the Neutralec Neutraliser that started out life as a solution to a carpet problem, and was found unexpectedly to be beneficial for people's health? (See page 113.) The dog that suddenly stopped barking (page 15) and the cows that were healthier and produced more milk (page 23) did not know that the geopathic stress had been fixed. How can the sceptics explain the dramatic drop in motor accidents at a traffic black-spot (page 16) after some quartz pillars were placed near the road? The study by

Ann and Roy Procter (page 7) allowed for the placebo effect and still produced impressive results. Alf Riggs' uncanny ability to identify exactly where a cancer would be located is difficult to explain (page 77). All this suggests that there is something going on that has some validity.

Geopathic energies challenge our current understanding of how bodies work and what affects them. Michael Shallis in *The Electric Shock Book* remarks:

> Electricity and magnetism can be seen as the intermediary between the material world and the ethereal world, touching us physically but also linking us to other realms of the totality of creation. It is through electromagnetism that we can perceive the subtle forces that operate in those intangible regions.

Including knowledge of geopathic energies in our understanding of illness requires a much more holistic view of man: one which takes into account the role of ch'i, the subtle bodies, the meridians, the chakras, yin and yang. This view of man sees the importance of harmony and balance within the body, and also between people and their environment. Some of the frameworks from quantum physics may also be useful in deepening our understanding.

These unseen energies help to remind us that we are more than just physical bodies with a mind, that we have dimensions beyond that which our normal senses can understand. We have an energy presence that can be disturbed by other energy presences, and we ignore this fact at our peril.

This book is predominantly concerned with geopathic stress, but three related topics:

- Electromagnetic pollution
- Sick building syndrome
- Feng shui

are covered in a brief way here.

APPENDIX 1

MAN-MADE ELECTROMAGNETIC POLLUTION

It is clearly unrealistic to try to go back to a time when mankind did not use electricity and magnetism, but it is important that this area of growing concern is fully investigated. X rays were found to be dangerous if unwisely used, and so adequate safeguards had to be developed for harnessing their potential for good and minimising their possibility of harm. The same process has to be gone through for electrical appliances and communication systems. In earlier centuries both magnetism and electricity were thought to be caused by fluids. This view is now clearly recognised as incorrect, but this does not mean that the current scientific understanding of electricity and magnetism is totally correct.

Undoubtedly, in some areas our health has improved dramatically, because of improved heating, sewage disposal and hygiene. We now live longer, and some diseases have become uncommon. Many of these improvements have come about partly as a result of the development of electricity. Yet the possible negative effects of this dependence on electricity are just beginning to show. These negative effects of electricity are usually referred to as electromagnetic pollution or electromagnetic smog.

Without electricity and magnetism we would not have television, hi-fi systems, radios, computers, telephones, electric lights and many other things. A power cut reminds us all very quickly of how dependent our lives have become on electricity. There are also many magnets in our homes, although we are largely unaware of their existence. Fridge doors generally use magnets to create a firm closure. Hi-fi speakers and telephone earpieces are dependent on magnets for their proper functioning. Many burglar alarms use magnets as part of their warning system. The brown strips on the back of credit cards are magnetic. Computer disks, videotapes and audiotapes contain tiny magnets.

Many of our body processes have an electrical or magnetic component to them (see chapter 6), so it would not be surprising if man-made electromagnetic energies affected the body in some way. We know that electromagnetic waves do not stop at the skin but penetrate the body. In fact people act all the time like a receiver. This can be shown very simply using a television set. If the normal aerial is removed, the picture deteriorates. If a finger is placed over the aerial socket, the picture immediately improves. Reception is not as good as with the proper aerial, but this does show that the television waves in the air can be conducted through the physical body and into the television set. Even without being connected to the television these waves are present. The transmitters are transmitting all the time, so we are experiencing television and radio waves whether we are in a building or in the street or out in the countryside.

Electrical Power

Electricity, produced by power stations, is distributed via power lines to homes, factories and offices throughout the country. In the U.K. the power stations produce electricity at a voltage of 25,000 V (25 kV). The voltage is increased further by step-up transformers to 400 kV. Electricity at this voltage is carried by very large pylons with very good insulation, because it is potentially lethal. The reason these high voltages are used is that it allows electricity to be carried in the most efficient way possible, minimising heat and, therefore, energy loss.

Then as it nears towns, step-down transformer stations reduce the voltage to 132 kV. At this point smaller pylons or underground cables can carry the electricity. Then at substations the voltage is reduced even further. In the case of lines to residential houses this would be 230 V (110 volts in the USA). 230 v is used because it is a compromise between safety and efficient transportation of electricity within the home. It is possible to survive an electric shock from 230 volts, but not from anything higher. Once in homes the electricity travels via the ring main to the various sockets. This electricity can then be used to run washing machines, televisions, vacuum cleaners, video machines, central heating and hot water systems and all the other appliances that are dependent on it.

Electrical Fields & Magnetic Fields

When an appliance is plugged into the socket, an electrical field exists even if it is not switched on. Unplugging the appliance will stop the electrical field existing in the cable of the appliance, but it will still exist in the wiring in the wall. Once the appliance is switched on both an electrical and a magnetic field exist. The electrical field flows along the cable and the magnetic field is at right angles to it. In a home the background magnetic field produced by wiring and mains appliances is typically 0.01-0.2 microtesla. Most concern is about exposure to fields greater than 0.4 microtesla. The distance from the source (appliances, wiring, etc.) markedly affects exposure to the magnetic field. People continue to be exposed to electromagnetic fields at work (computers, heating and industrial processes, etc.) and while travelling.

Power lines also produce electrical and magnetic fields. The strength of the electrical field gradually decreases the further away from the wires, but the magnetic field decreases more rapidly. Metal, trees, buildings and walls reduce the effect of electrical fields, but magnetic fields pass through most surfaces. Where the high-voltage cables are underground, the magnetic field at ground level is much higher immediately above the cable than for the equivalent overhead power line. The magnetic field from the overhead line decreases less rapidly than that from the underground line the further away from the cable. When power lines are buried they do not produce an electrical field at the surface. (18)

Radiation

Ionising radiation is able to split apart atoms and molecules, whereas non-ionising radiation is not. The fact that ionising radiation is known to do this immediately gives an understanding of how devastating this type of radiation can be. Nuclear weapons make use of this for their effect. Medical X-rays also involve small, carefully controlled doses.

Non-ionising radiation includes the spectrum of ultraviolet, visible light, infrared, microwave (MW), radio frequency (RF), and extremely low frequency waves (ELF). Microwaves are used for satellite communication, radar detection devices and telemetry (remote switching of water pumps, machinery, sewage works, electricity sub stations, etc.) as well as in microwave cookers. Microwave radiation is absorbed near the skin surface.

Radio frequency radiation (from television, radio broadcasts and mobile phone transmissions) may be absorbed throughout the body. At high enough intensities both microwaves and radio waves will damage tissue through heating. This is usually only a problem when equipment is malfunctioning

Extremely Low Frequency Waves

Faulty microwave ovens can cook people as well as food. People die from electric shocks from wrongly wired appliances. These problems are well recognised. It is the non-thermal effects from properly functioning equipment which are much more in dispute, particularly the level at which the effects become harmful.

The main concern in terms of safety for the general public is with extremely low frequency waves. Extremely low frequency fields produce non-ionizing radiation from 1 Hz to 300 Hz. These are produced by power lines, electrical wiring, and electrical equipment. This type of radiation does not split atoms and molecules. Current scientific knowledge does not provide us with any understanding of how these ELFs could damage living organisms, so many scientists are unwilling to accept the possibility that this could happen.

The Safety Of ELFs

In 1992 the UK National Radiological Protection Board reviewed the evidence on electromagnetic fields and the risk of cancer and criticised the methodology of many of the studies. In the report it argued that many of the studies supporting such a link were flawed in some way. The Board urged that many more rigorous studies were necessary, but went on to say:

> It cannot be concluded either that electromagnetic fields have no effect on the physiology of cells, even if the fields are weak, or that they produce effects that would, in other circumstances, be regarded as suggestive of potential carcinogenicity.

Some years later the Canadian government produced a report:

Heath Effects and Exposure Guidelines Related to Extremely Low Frequency Electric and Magnetic Fields - An Overview. The Federal Provincial Territorial Radiation Protection Committee (FPTRPC) established an ELF Working Group to review the scientific literature in relation to health effects of exposure to ELF radiation. The first report was published in 1998 and updated in 2002. The report includes a 'position statement for the general public'. On cancer the report concludes:

> Epidemiological studies have not established an association between exposure to power-frequency EMFs and the development of cancer in adults. The evidence associating cancers in children with exposure to power-frequency EMFs remains inconclusive.

The report also does not believe that the case for the wider damage of ELFs has been proved:

> Based on the available scientific evidence to date, the Federal Provincial Territorial Radiation Protection Committee (FPTRPC) concludes that adverse health effects from exposure to power-frequency EMFs, at levels normally encountered in homes, schools and offices, have not been established.

This seems to be the view of most of the scientific and medical community – ELFs have no health implications except possibly for childhood leukaemia. Yet the concern of the general public refuses to go away. Many people can give anecdotal evidence of problems with EMF's, and an improvement in health when these are negated in some way. The story of how the Neutralec Neutraliser, a device to counteract problems with carpet pile, (see page 113) came to be used to counteract electromagnetic fields gives some credence that this is not all a placebo effect. In their literature Neutralec (28) talk of the case of a man who only had epileptic fits when in the vicinity of a bedside tea maker, or immediately beneath it in the room below. Twelve months after having the Neutralec fitted, the man had had no further fits.

The London Hazards Centre (25) also believes that non-ionising radiation may cause problems. In its booklet *Sick Building Syndrome* it says:

> Electromagnetic radiation at either ionising or non-ionising frequencies is virtually impossible to measure accurately in the office and at the low levels concerned. Different frequencies need different methods of measurement, and at extremely low frequencies the instruments themselves can interfere with and distort the fields that they are measuring.

The same booklet also says:

> ...depending on the layout of the room, people who spend no time at all at a VDU may actually have higher exposure than those working on the screen: many VDUs emit more radiation from the side and back than from the front.

De-Kun Li, a reproductive epidemiologist at the Kaiser Foundation Research Institute in Oakland, California, USA, measured the exposure of pregnant women to magnetic fields. His team studied 1063 women who were in the first ten weeks of pregnancy. Each woman spent a day wearing a meter that measured the magnetic field levels every ten seconds. They found that women who were exposed to a peak level of 1.6 microteslas or greater were nearly twice as likely to miscarry as women who were not exposed to such strong fields. *Epidemiology* 2002;13:9-20

It could be that ELFs do contribute to many health problems, but this effect is not found on statistical analysis because ELF exposure is only part of a whole complex of factors that are not amenable to easy analysis. Another possibility is that ELFs are affecting the health of everyone, so that it is not possible to find the effect in epidemiological studies. The increase in allergies, the development of new diseases and the levels of unhappiness found in the general population may be indicators that the majority of people are being affected by EMF exposure to some degree. This proposition is difficult to test. It is impossible to find a population that has a low exposure to ELFs but shares all the other characteristics of a modern society. Where there is low ELF exposure, diet and life style are likely to be very different.

Professor Denis L. Henshaw of Bristol University (19) believes that radiation levels from power lines may interact with particles of air pollution so that exposure to air pollution is increased for people near by. This could be an indirect way of power lines leading to serious health problems.

To complicate matters even further, it may well be that only some people are susceptible to problems from EMFs. Even these people are not necessarily sensitive to all EMFs. In a study entitled *Electrical Sensitivities in Allergy Patients* (*Clin Ecol* 1987) Dr V.S. Choy and his colleagues found that some of their allergy patients were sensitive to specific frequencies rather than to specific intensities. They found that the mechanism for switching off these sensitivities was the same as they would use for foods and chemicals.

Reducing Exposure To Electromagnetic Pollution

Erring on the side of safety it is probably advisable to reduce the amount of exposure to electromagnetic pollution particularly while sleeping. Many people have found that simple changes can lead to dramatic improvements in health.

Several of my clients have found that they start sleeping better if they either stop using an electric blanket, or at least unplug it at the socket at night. Remember that the electric field is still there when the blanket is plugged in but not switched on. Of course, many people have electric clocks and tea making machines very close to their heads while they are sleeping, and this may be inadvisable at least for susceptible people. It is very simple to check whether removing these for a time makes any difference. Using mechanical clocks rather than electric clocks in the bedroom is a sensible precaution. Powerwatch (29) recommends that electric clocks and tea making equipment should be kept at least one metre (approximately 3 feet) from the sleeping position. It has also been suggested that metal bedsprings can amplify negative energy, so it may be worth considering using a mattress of a different construction.

Wearing mechanical rather than electronic watches can also make a difference for some people. Re-organising the way that computers and word processors are placed in a work environment can have a significant impact on health, particularly if it is remembered that there may be more radiation from the back of the computer than from the front. If the house is next to an electricity substation it may be as well to organise sleeping arrangements so that everyone, and particularly children, sleep as far away from it as possible. Erring on the side of caution may be a wise thing to do.

Protective Devices

There are also lots of devices on the market offering personal protection against electromagnetic pollution. Some of the devices mentioned in chapter 9 also offer protection against electromagnetic pollution, but some of the manufacturers make devices specifically to counteract it. Pulsors (see page 130), EMF Life Transformers (see page 129), portable Neutralec Neutralisers (see page 113) and portable Geomacks (see page 111) may be helpful. There does not seem to be one single device that everyone finds works for them, so it may be necessary to try different ones. Fortunately most come with a money-back guarantee.

Using Essences

Some essences have been designed to counteract problems with electromagnetic pollution. The Alaskan Essences Guardian remedy (01) can be used to counteract both geopathic and EMF problems. The Australian Bush Flower Essences (04) offer the Electro Essence that:

> Greatly relieves fear and distress associated with earth, electrical and electromagnetic radiation. It helps to bring one into balance with the natural rhythms of the earth.

Degaussing The Body

Degaussing the body (see page 130) can be useful to counteract electromagnetic pollution as well as geopathic stress.

The mother of one of my clients commented that she had experienced headaches since going back to work. These only occurred on the days she worked. She was convinced it was because she was working with VDU's, but did not know what to do about it, other than give up her job. I suggested she should try degaussing once a week for a trial period. Two months later she told me that she had not had a single headache since she had started doing this. She was completely mystified as to how this could possibly work, but delighted that she could continue with her job without the headaches.

Another client told me his eczema was getting worse again. He had bought a computer and was spending a lot of time using it. Once he started degaussing himself with his wife's hair drier his eczema started to improve again.

Many people experience another positive benefit of doing this in that they become less 'addicted' to television. They now find it easier to switch off the television, the video games or their computer. People who are prone to static electric shocks usually find this procedure beneficial too. Here again the benefit is temporary so that the procedure needs to be repeated on a regular basis.

****

Many people are convinced that electromagnetic pollution is damaging the quality of their lives leading to a whole series of problems including cancers. Most of the scientific community thinks that the link between non-ionising radiation and ill health is non-existent or far from proven. Only time will tell which view is correct.

With the increasing use of electricity in the form of computers, power lines, televisions and so on, the total electromagnetic load on people has increased. This may make many individuals susceptible to much lower levels of geopathic stress. These people will exhibit symptoms sooner from a given level of exposure to geopathic energies than if they were not also exposed to electromagnetic pollution.

Appendix 2

SICK BUILDING SYNDROME

Definition & Symptoms

The term 'sick building syndrome' (SBS) is generally related to the physical environment of a building. The World Health Organisation defines sick building syndrome as:

> ...a syndrome of complaints covering non-specific feelings of malaise the onset of which is associated with occupancy of certain buildings

Common symptoms for the individual include tiredness, confusion, headaches, flu like symptoms, skin rashes, problems with the eyes, nose, throat and chest (often involving a feeling of dryness in the mucus membranes), dizziness and nausea. This can lead to absenteeism, reduced efficiency, lowered morale and increased staff turnover.

Sick building syndrome can be seen as a reaction to a cluster of problems often found in modern buildings. In some buildings the air conditioning is not maintained to a high enough standard, allowing moulds and bacteria to build up in the air conditioning ducting. Lack of adequate ventilation, glare from lights, ozone and chemical fumes from photocopiers and computers can make people feel unwell. Volatile chemicals from carpets, chipboard, plastics, etc. can all cause problems. Buildings that are too hot or too cold, and exposure to perfume from other employees can distress and dissatisfy employees.

People feeling that they have no control over their environment may also exacerbate the physical problems. For example, employees cannot adjust the temperature in sealed, centrally-controlled, air-conditioned buildings to suit themselves. This leads people to feel powerless, a major source of stress in its own right. In addition, many modern open-plan buildings offer little individual privacy. Some buildings have very little, if any, natural light. This may lead to disturbance in the natural daily rhythms of the body when it no longer has the stimulus from the natural environment.

In 1995 the Inland Revenue decided to demolish a 19-storey office where half of the 2000 staff had suffered frequently from flu-like symptoms for more than 5 years, even though biocides had been used to counteract the proliferation of bacteria etc. in the water reservoir of the air-conditioning system (*The Perils of Progress* by John Ashton).

The Evidence

Some scientists and employers are sceptical about the existence of sick building syndrome. The UK Health & Safety Executive (Local Authority Circular 75/1) definition reflects this:

> SBS is a term used to describe a building in which the occupants experience a range of symptoms causing discomfort and a sense of being unwell, rather than specific illnesses. These buildings are typically modern offices which have mechanical ventilation or air conditioning. It is a complex problem and much of the evidence for it is inconclusive and circumstantial. Both physical and psychological causes have been suggested.

A F Marmot et al published a study in *Occupational and Environmental Medicine* (2006;63:283-289). Their subjects were 4052 office-based government employees aged 42–62 years working in 44 buildings. They looked at the physical environment of the workplace and self-reported symptoms. Respondents were asked if they had experienced in the last 14 days any of ten symptoms commonly associated with sick building syndrome. The symptoms included headaches, dry itchy eyes and dry throats. One in seven of the men, and almost one in five of the women reported experiencing at least five of the symptoms. The buildings were also assessed for temperature, lighting intensity, levels of airborne pollution, etc.

The study did not find a link between the usual sick building factors and employee sickness and absenteeism:

> The physical environment of office buildings appears to be less important than features of the psychosocial work environment [including high job demands and low support] in explaining differences in the prevalence of symptoms.

Professor Alan Hedge, of the Department of Design & Environmental Analysis at Cornell University, USA, offers an explanation of why it may be difficult to establish a link. In a paper he presented at the 1st Asian Indoor Air Quality Seminar in China in 1996 he said:

> Questionnaires usually collect data on workers' perceptions of environmental conditions and health over extended periods of time, such as one month, 3 months, 1 year, whereas measures of environmental conditions seldom are taken over such extensive periods. Moreover, such measurements normally are not taken for each individual location in a building. Thus, it is perhaps not surprising that little association between self-reported symptoms and measured IAQ [indoor air quality] has been found.

In his conclusion to this paper he says:

> Research shows that IAQ problems and reports of the SBS [sick building syndrome] generally are not caused simply by exposure to poor IAQ, but rather they occur because of the combined effects of various physical environment and non-environmental factors. IAQ complaints and the SBS are the outcome of complex processes,

initiated by a set of stressful multiple risks which create personal strain.

One of the problems for any analysis in this area is that buildings that are bad physically often also have managers who have a disrespectful attitude to their work force. It can be difficult then to isolate the symptoms that are solely attributable to the building itself.

This is undoubtedly a complex area, which is further complicated by the often contrasting demands of employers and employees. It is clear that if geopathic stress is included as one of the components contributing to SBS, analysis of the situation becomes even more complex. It may well be that GS is a causative factor that is often overlooked.

APPENDIX 3

FENG SHUI

Feng shui, originating in China, is based on the observation that people are affected by their environment, and that it is possible to influence how people feel and behave by considering and perhaps changing the environment in which they live. The term 'feng shui' means 'wind-water', and the aim of the feng shui practitioner is to enhance the flow of energies in the landscape, integrating people, buildings and the landscape into a harmonious whole. Feng Shui experts believe that when this is done good health, happiness and prosperity will result.

Ch'i

Central to feng shui is the concept of ch'i. Feng shui practices are designed to heal the flow of ch'i, so that it moves freely without violence or stagnation. As we have already seen (page 64), ch'i is the primary subtle energy of the universe, flowing into man and becoming his own personal ch'i. Sarah Rossbach explains in *Feng Shui*:

> Ch'i is a life essence, a motivating force. It animates all things. Ch'i determines the height of mountains, the quality of blooms, the extent of potential fulfilment. Without ch'i, trees will not blossom, rivers will not flow, man will not be.

Yin & Yang

In considering the harmonious flow of ch'i, the Chinese draw on the concepts of yin and yang. Ch'i energy is both yin and yang. Yin is often depicted as female energy, and yang as male energy. Heaven is seen as being male and the earth as being female. What is between has to develop a balance between male and female, so that harmony and balance can ensue. As well as being male, yang is seen as being active, light and expansive, whereas yin is seen as being passive, dark and receptive. Too much 'male' energy is harmful, just as too much 'female' energy is. Harmony is achieved when yin and yang are in balance. Yin and yang are not seen as being in conflict: they depend on each other.

This balance is not static, although it is often depicted in this way. It is a dynamic fluctuating balance leading to growth, change and harmony. A static balance would lead to rigidity and death without renewal. Life is seen as being a continuous cycle of yang and yin. Death leads to new life. Rest leads to renewal and new activity. Night is followed by day; winter is followed by summer. These changes are part of the natural and harmonious cycle of life. Although at any one time yin or yang may predominate, over time they maintain harmony.

These changes form part of a complementary cycle, but sometimes yang or yin predominates inappropriately. Excess yang may result in frenetic activity with no time for rest and renewal. There is excess heat and growth without the cooling effect of yin. Excessive yin results in stagnation and sluggishness without the stimulation and fire of yang.

Landscapes can be classified as representing either yin or yang. A yin landscape is flat, but not totally flat; a yang landscape is mountainous, but not too steep. The extremes would exhibit an excess of that quality. The concept of yin and yang can also be applied to many other situations. Frantic economic activity, for example, can be seen as excessive yang. This is, almost inevitably, counterbalanced by a recession, excessive yin. Climates too can be seen as displaying excess yin or excess yang. A hot dry climate would have excessive yang, whereas a wet cool climate would be showing too much yin.

These imbalances within the environment or within the person can lead to physical illness. Each type of illness is related to whether yin or yang are in excess. Yang illnesses are characterised by heat and activity, yin illnesses by congestion and dampness. Where ch'i does not flow, paralysis results. From a feng shui point of view imbalances within the individual will often mirror imbalances within that person's environment. It is felt that the person will find it difficult, if not impossible, to attain harmony within themselves, if there is a lack of harmony in the environment (excessive yin or excessive yang).

So it is vitally important that the flow of ch'i is harmonious. It is not a luxury, but a necessity for people to live happy, healthy and harmonious lives. Harmonious ch'i encourages growth, well-being, abundance and good fortune.

There can be an absence of Ch'i leading to barrenness and lack of success, because the flow of ch'i has been blocked in some way. More frequently, ch'i is flowing, but there is an imbalance in the yin and yang qualities of it. If there is too much yin energy, then there will be slowness and a lack of vitality, so this has to be counterbalanced by increasing the yang qualities in the landscape. The flow of ch'i can also exhibit too much yang, so that growth is uncontrolled and unbalanced, without attention being paid to nurturing and rest. Here there is too much yang energy, so the yin qualities of the landscape need to be enhanced.

Feng Shui

Feng Shui almost certainly grew out of the recognition that man tends to prosper in certain environments: where there is sunshine, but not too much heat; where there is rain and water, but not floods and damp. In other words man survives and prospers when there is some harmonious balance within the landscape and the climate.

Sarah Rossbach writes in *Feng Shui*:

> Despite its pragmatic aspect, feng shui is in a sense a rosetta stone linking man and his environment, ancient ways and modern life. It interprets the language articulated by natural forms and phenomena, by man-made buildings and symbols, and by the continual workings of the universe, including moon phases and star alignments. Feng shui is the key to understanding the silent dialogue between man and nature, whispered through a cosmic breath or spirit--ch'i..... If ch'i is misguided, man's life and luck might falter. Man feels and is affected by ch'i, though he may not know it.

Building Considerations

Ideally the landscape is assessed before any building takes place, so that buildings can be located in the most propitious way. This takes into account the natural flow of ch'i within the landscape, and also the way in which the landscape will be changed by the construction of the building. If the landscape has a very yang quality, then the house ideally would be situated where any yin qualities are present. So, for example, in a mountainous area, the house would be ideally situated in a valley. The plot should be square or rectangular, with the building facing south to make maximum use of the sun. The ideal building also has a regular shape to it and once again is often square or rectangular. Because of economic and practical considerations, this is not always possible, so remedial action may be necessary even with new buildings. The practitioner may work both on the house itself and on the landscape in which the building is situated.

Improving The Landscape

If it is not possible to choose the ideal location for a building, then it may be possible to alter the landscape. This allows ch'i to flow more smoothly, and yang and yin to achieve some degree of balance. Sometimes the shape of hills and the direction of streams is altered to make the flow of energy healthier. Land may be built up or lowered according to the need to harmonise the flow of energy. Where the land is very flat, soft hills will be added. Where the land is very steep, an attempt will be made to round and soften it, reducing abrupt changes of direction. Straight roads and rivers are to be avoided, as they conduct ch'i too quickly and have too much yang. Trees will often be planted in particular places. They enhance the correct flow of ch'i and also protect against harsh winds.

Water & Feng Shui

Water is seen as symbolising money, because it is essential for the production of rice. A house with a view of water is much sought after. Businesses also favour a view of water for similar reasons. It is said that the Hong Kong and Shanghai Bank helped the government with various developments in order to safeguard the view of Victoria Harbour from their building. Where a stream runs through a property this can be auspicious, but if the water flows too quickly it can cause money to leave too. A feng shui practitioner might advise that the flow of a stream or river needs to be changed, so that water flows more slowly; otherwise money, health and prosperity may flow through the building rather than being retained within it. However, if the building is located on a pointed promontory, there will be nothing to hold the money in. A garden pond also needs to be carefully sited: close enough to the building to enhance ch'i, but not too close to be a potential danger. Stagnant or polluted water, known as 'sha', may also cause problems for the inhabitants of the building.

Nearly all of these changes can be seen as making good sense in practical terms. A very straight river is liable to flooding. A house on a flat plain is exposed mercilessly to the elements. A pond or stream too close to a building can undermine the foundations and cause problems with dampness. It is not sensible to live close to polluted water. Even for those who do not accept the concepts of yin, yang and ch'i, the recommendations of the feng shui expert often make sense.

Improving The Building

Even if a building is situated ideally in the landscape, the interior of the building can undermine this good fortune and positive flow of ch'i. Buildings themselves may be modified. A building's entrance is particularly important, because this is symbolically where ch'i enters. It needs to be open enough to allow the smooth entry of ch'i, but enclosed enough to protect the inhabitants. In other words it needs to embody a balance of yin and yang qualities. The Hong Kong/USA Asian Trade Center in Oakland California was altered on the advice of a feng shui expert. A central column was removed, because it was said to block the flow of ch'i at the entrance to the complex.

New windows may be put in or corners smoothed. Furniture may be moved to a more pleasing arrangement or may be removed altogether. It is felt that beds and desks should always be placed where it is possible to see the door, partly to avoid being surprised by someone entering unseen.

Using Artefacts To Correct Imbalances

Mirrors, wind chimes, bells, flutes, mobiles, stones, and statues are used to improve ch'i. Each type of object has its own characteristic way of influencing ch'i. Placing is of vital importance. Several doors aligned in a row are said to encourage ch'i to move too quickly, so a mobile or wind chime may be hung from one of the doorframes to slow this flow. Plants are used to help ch'i to move more freely and so are particularly useful in an area where ch'i tends to be stagnant.

Much of the thinking behind using colours and objects to enhance the flow of ch'i takes into account their symbolic nature. For example, bright lights strategically placed are seen to represent the sun and its positive flow of yang energy, countering too much dark (yin) energy. A practitioner might consider placing additional lights (yang) in a dark (excess yin) hallway. Green is used to stimulate growth and yellow to represent the sun. Plants remind people of nature and growth. Flutes symbolise safety and good will, because they were used in the past to announce good news. Heavy objects are used to stabilise ch'i. Mirrors are used to reflect negative ch'i. Sarah Rossbach describes mirrors as:

> ... the all-purpose remedy... the aspirin of feng shui' *Feng Shui*

Mirrors can be also be used to balance badly proportioned rooms, re-directing ch'i more positively and counteracting stagnant spots.

The right object in the wrong place will not do its job effectively and may even damage the flow of ch'i. In looking at an area it is always important to consider the balance of yin and yang. Adding items with yin qualities to an area that has an excess of yin energy will further unbalance the flow of ch'i and increase the distress of the occupants.

In her book *Interior Design With Feng Shui* Sarah Rossbach makes an interesting comment on computers:

> According to modern feng shui experts, computers affect ch'i. Computers can be good, enlivening and stimulating to the office. They can raise wisdom and knowledge. The computer worker, however, should face the door or he or she will suffer from stress and neurosis after a while.

Feng shui is concerned with the form and shape of the landscape and buildings and the way in which this moulds and distorts ch'i energy. Feng shui philosophy very firmly locates man in his environment: it is not possible to consider his health without looking at his environment.

Feng Shui & Geopathic Stress

It is clear that there are a lot of cross-links between geopathic stress and feng shui. Both disciplines are concerned with the influence of the environment on people. Both are concerned with the energy of places. Both use artefacts to alter and improve this. Some of these artefacts are even the same.

Nicholas Fernee In *Wind and Water* (*International Journal of Alternative and Complementary Medicine*, August 1993) says:

> At a more general level the findings of geopathic stress advocates ..... have confirmed the dramatic effect upon health that underground water can have, known in Feng Shui as Sha, or 'noxious vapours', this being an example of negative Chi.

In spite of all this overlap and common ground correcting geopathic energies does not automatically correct ch'i, nor does following feng shui precepts correct all geopathic energies. To some extent the two disciplines are looking at different types of energy, although there is much common ground. There are clearly overlaps between the two, and it could be argued that for a full appraisal of the energy of a site, it would be wise to consult both a feng shui expert and a geopathic stress practitioner. The geopathic stress expert would concentrate on correcting the negative earth energies, while the Feng Shui practitioner would concentrate on bringing harmony and prosperity to the site.

APPENDIX 4

EARTH ENERGY ESSENCES

See page 8 for more information on these.

The Earth Energies come in 30 ml bottles for dispensing. They are also available as a small test kit for testing using kinesiology or dowsing. Although produced from the energies in Cornwall (England), they seem to benefit people wherever they live.

BALANCE is for the times when we need more balance in our lives; when we find our energies easily disturbed and drained by other people and by our environment. Over-sensitivity, fragility and moodiness could indicate a need for this remedy.

This energy was collected from a rock protruding out into the rushing stream that runs through the magical Trevaylor Woods (west Cornwall, UK). It was a damp and misty day in winter with water dripping from the leaves, ferns and mosses which grew everywhere in great profusion.

COMFORT is for times when energy and a willingness to persist are hard to find. It brings a feeling of gentle warmth into our lives. Feeling lost, vulnerable, defenceless and abandoned could indicate a need for this remedy.

This energy was collected at Godrevey (west Cornwall, UK), standing on a cliff overlooking the sea. The cliffs were carpeted with blue and yellow flowers. Although it was early June it was cold and overcast, but the underside of the lower clouds shone with a promise of better things to come. The sea seemed timeless as the waves broke on the shore. It was early evening and there were still people about, but they seemed frozen in their activity: two men fishing off one of the rocks, surfers in the sea and couples sitting in their cars and gazing into the distance.

ENERGY & REALISM gives energy and stamina. It helps to bring realism to our activities, so that tasks can be started and accomplished in a balanced manner. Both obsessive and unfocussed behaviour become less extreme. Feeling frantic and indecisive could indicate a need for this remedy.

This energy was collected by perching on a hump of granite, partly surrounded by spring water emerging from rock-strewn moorland between Bosigran Cliffs and the towering Carn Calver (west Cornwall, UK). This was collected on the same day as "Need", when the earlier bright skies had clouded over, giving the wind even more bite.

INNER WISDOM is for times when we are lacking discernment and discipline in our lives. We may feel that life is chaotic and uncertain, even while we present an air of power, wisdom and competence to others. The inner life does not correspond with the outer world's perception. Often our energy levels will appear to others to be high, but this mirage is maintained at great cost to ourselves.

This energy was collected from a wide fissure in a massive rock outcrop on the north coast of Cornwall between Zennor and Morvah (west Cornwall, UK). It was a cold, bright day. From this place high on the cliffs, the long Atlantic swells could be seen and heard breaking over the rocks below, and gulls soared over the cliffs.

NEED is to help us to distinguish between needs and wants; it gives the quiet security that our needs *will* be met. Feelings of jealousy, frustration, disappointment, insecurity, fearfulness and an inability to settle and be still could indicate a need for this remedy.

This energy was collected from a partly ruinous stone circle on Bosporthennis Moor to the west of Mulfra Hill (west Cornwall, UK). It is thought by some to be the remains of a hut circle rather than a true stone circle, but has a great feeling of "rightness". The bright sunshine failed to warm the bitter March wind blasting across the moor.

PAIN is for pain, bewilderment and a sense of isolation, when even feeling these emotions seems to demand too much energy. Feelings of weakness and helplessness could indicate a need for this remedy.

This energy was collected from the seaward end of the Cot Valley (west Cornwall, UK). The valley is steep sided and rocky, opening to the sea between high cliffs where the stream runs into a small cove famed for its smoothly rounded boulders. On a day of seemingly interminable rain, with the land shrouded in mist, when we arrived to collect this energy the sky lightened and rain stopped. I had established several days before that the new essence would be called "Pain" and, as I climbed up towards the site, I was feeling it, having squashed my toe under a door the previous day. The place I wanted turned out to be a craggy point overlooking the Brisons Rock, where the swell heaved and broke fitfully.

SPACE is for times when we need physical, emotional, mental or spiritual space. When things press in on us so that we cannot think clearly or see our way forward, this essence helps to create the possibility for much needed change. It helps us to find vision and continuity within our roots. Feeling overwhelmed or inadequate could indicate a need for this remedy.

This essence was collected from high on the sides of Carn Calver (west Cornwall, UK). A strong wind blustered off the wide Atlantic to the west and open moorland stretched to distant carns on the other sides. The area was strewn with lumps of granite tumbled from the summit like some giant's toy building blocks. A great weather-sculpted slab of rock provided the focus of the energy.

These can be bought directly from the author (36) or from the secure online shop at www.lifeworkpotential.com.

REFERENCES

John Ashton
The Perils Of Progress
Zen Books Ltd., 1999, ISBN 185649697X

Kathe Bachler
Earth Radiation
Wordmasters Ltd., 1989, ISBN 095141510 7

Christopher Bird
The Divining Hand
Whitford Press, 1993, ISBN 0924608161

Barbara Ann Brennan
Hands of Light
Bantam, 1988, ISBN 0553345397

Canadian Government: The Federal Provincial Territorial
Radiation Protection Committee (FPTRPC)
Heath Effects and Exposure Guidelines Related to Extremely
Low Frequency Electric and Magnetic Fields - An Overview
Available for download as a PDF document at www.bccdc.org

Deepak Chopra
Quantum Healing
Bantam,1990, ISBN 055317332 4

Ray V.S. Choy, Jean A. Monroe & Cyril W. Smith
Electrical Sensitivity in Allergy Patients
Clinical Ecology, Volume IV, Number 3, 1986

David Cowan
Safe As Houses?
Currently out of print but can be read or downloaded from
www.leyman.demon.co.uk

John Davidson
Radiation
Random House, 2004, ISBN 0852071809

Paul Devereux
Places of Power
Cassell, 1999, ISBN 0713727659

Steve Eabry
Biogenic Magnetite in Humans
International Journal of Alternative & Complementary Medicine,
January 1993

Nicholas Fernee
Wind and Water: a Brief Introduction to Feng Shui
International Journal of Alternative & Complementary Medicine,
August 1993
J Havelock Fidler
Ley Lines
Turnstone Press Ltd., 1985, ISBN 0855001739

David Furlong
Earth Energies
Piatkus, 2003, ISBN 0749923679

Richard Gerber, M.D.
Vibrational Medicine
Bear & Company Publishing, 2001, ISBN 187981584

Rolf Gordon
Are You Sleeping In A Safe Place?
Dulwich Health Society, 2005, ISBN 095140170X

Tom Graves
The Dowser's Workbook
Sterling, 1990, ISBN 0806973986

Tom Graves & Janet Hoult (Ed)
The Essential T.C. Lethbridge
Arkana, 1988, 0140194045

Tom Graves
Needles of Stone Revisited
Gothic Image Publications. 1978. ISBN 0906362075
Now out of print but available as a free download from the
author's web site www.tomgraves.com.au

Julian Kenyon
Bio-energetic Regulatory Medicine
International Journal of Alternative & Complementary Medicine,
January 1994

Drew Leder
"Spooky Action At A Distance": Physics, Psi, and Distant
Healing
Journal of Alternative And Complementary Medicine
Vol 11, Number 5, 2005, pp 923-930

London Hazards Centre
Sick Building Syndrome
London Hazards Centre, 1990, ISBN 0948974060

Patrick MacManaway
Dowsing For Health
Anness Publishing Limited, 2001, ISBN 1843094355

Electromagnetic Fields and The Risk of Cancer
National Radiological Protection Board, 1992, ISBN 0859513467

Alasdair Philips
Living With Electricity
Powerwatch U.K., c/o 2 Tower Road, Sutton, Ely, Cambs., CB6
2QA

William Philpott
International Journal of Alternative & Complementary Medicine,
July 1992

Roy and Ann Procter
Healing Sick Houses
Gateway, 2000, ISBN 0 717129926

Sarah Rossbach
Feng Shui
Rider, 1992, ISBN 0712617620

Sarah Rossbach
Interior Design with Feng Shui
Rider, 1991, ISBN 0712614893

Michael Shallis
The Electric Shock Book
Souvenir Press, 1988, ISBN 028562827

Dr C W Smith
High-Sensitivity Biosensors And Weak Environment Stimuli
International Industrial Biotechnology, April/May 1986

David V Tansley
Radionics Interface With The Ether Fields
C.W. Daniel Co., Ltd., 1986, ISBN 0850321298

Jane Thurnell-Read
Geopathic Stress
International Journal of Alternative & Complementary Medicine,
April 1994

Jane Thurnell-Read
Health Kinesiology: The Muscle Testing System That Talks To
the Body
Life-Work Potential, 2002, ISBN 0954243900

Jane Thurnell-Read
Verbal Questioning Skills For Kinesiologists
Life-Work Potential, 2006, ISBN 0954243919

USEFUL ADDRESSES

(01) Alaskan Flower Essence Project
PO Box 1369
Homer, AK 99603
USA
Tel: 907-235-2188
Fax: 907-235-2777
Email: research@alaskanessences.com
www.alaskanessences.com

(02) American Society of Dowsers
P.O. Box 24
Danville, VT 05828
USA
Tel: 802-684-3417
Fax: 802-626-2565
Email: asd@dowsers.org
www.dowsers.org

(03) Applied Energetic Wisdom (Tony G. Mills)
PO Box 51625
London, SE8 3YT
UK
Tel: 084 5345 4374 or 07791 549 193
Email: info@rednineharmoniser.com
www.rednineharmoniser.com

(04) Australian Bush Flower Essences
45 Booralie Road, Terrey Hills
NSW, 2084
Australia
Tel: 02 9450 1388
Fax: 02 9450 2866
Email: info@ausflowers.com.au
www.ausflowers.com.au

(05) Sylvia Bennett
Taddlestone, Slapton
Devon, TQ7 2QT
UK
01548 580989
Email: sylvia@fengshui-living.com
www.fengshui-living.com

(06) Giulia Boden
Sycamore Cottage, Chalford Hill
Midway, Stroud
Gloucestershire, GL6 8EN
UK
Tel: 01453 889184
Email: giuliadence@yahoo.co.uk
www.hk4health.co.uk/geocourse.htm

(07) British Society Of Dowsers
National Dowsing Centre
2 St Ann's Road, Malvern
Worcestershire. WR14 4RG
UK
Tel & Fax: 01684 576969.
Email: info@britishdowsers.org
www.britishdowsers.org

(08) Canadian Society Of Dowsers
7- 800 Queenston Road, Suite 152,
Stoney Creek
ON L8G 1A7
Canada
Tel: 888 588 8958
www.canadiandowsers.org

(09) Central Life Harmony
Josephine Harris
16 Victor Road
Colchester, CO1 2LU
UK
Tel: 01206 862177
Email: jobrambles@hotmail.com

(10) Creative Building Solutions
Chris Tivey
1 Wenlock Way
Maldon, Essex, CM9 5AE
UK
Tel: 01621 859272
Email: chris@creativebuildingsolutions.co.uk

(11) Dowsers Society of NSW (Australia)
www.divstrat.com.au/DSNSW/index.html

(12) Dowsing Society of Victoria Inc. (Australia)
www.dsv.org.au

(13) Dulwich Health Society and Rolf Gordon
130 Gipsy Hill
London, SE19 1PL
UK
Tel: 020 8670 5883
Fax: 020 8766 6616
www.dulwichhealth.co.uk

(14) The Feng Shui Society
377 Edgware Road
London W2 1BT
UK
Tel: 07050 289 200
Email: info@fengshuisociety.org.uk
www.fengshuisociety.org.uk

(15) Geomack
PO Box 369
Ramsgate
Kent, CT11 9YZ
UK
Tel: 01843 570.870
Fax: 01843 570.970
Email: sales@geomack.com
www.geomack.com

(16) Health Kinesiology (International) and Jimmy Scott Ph.D.
RR3 Hastings
Ontario, KOL 1YO
Canada
Tel: 705 696 3176
Email: hk@subtlenergy.com
www.subtlenergy.com

(17) Health Kinesiology UK
Tel: 08707 655980 (to find a practitioner)
Tel: 01246 862339 (to find a trainer
www.hk4health.co.uk

(18) Health Protection Agency Central Office (UK)
7th Floor, Holborn Gate
330 High Holborn
London, WC1V 7PP
UK
Tel: 020 7759 2700 / 2701
Fax: 020 7759 2733
www.hpa.org.uk

(19) Human Radiation Effects Group (University of Bristol)
H. H. Wills Physics Laboratory
Tyndall Avenue
Bristol, BS8 1TL
UK
Tel: 0117 926 0353
Fax: 0117 925 1723
www.electric-fields.bris.ac.uk

(20) Jordstralningscentrum (Sweden)
Tel +46-8 510 110 25
Email: jc@spray.se
www.jordstralningscentrum.nu

(21) Kinesiology Federation
PO Box 28908
Dalkeith, EH22 2YQ
UK
Tel: 08700 113545
Email: kfadmin@kinesiologyfederation.org
www.kinesiologyfederation.org

(22) Vivian Klein
Santa Rosa, California, USA
Tel: 707 538 8679
Fax: 707 538 3623
Email: viviklein@earthlink.net
Vivian also travels to Israel several times a year

(23)Gina Lazenby
The Healthy Home
P O Box 249, Keighley
West Yorkshire, BD20 8YN
UK
Tel: 07000 336 474
Email: bettersleep@thehealthyhome.com
www.thehealthyhome.com

(24) Sylvie Lenoir
3 Brookend Street
Ross-on-Wye
Herefordshire, HR9 7EG
UK
Tel: 01989 763 999
Email: sylvie.lenoir@btconnect.com

(25) London Hazards Centre
Headland House
308 Gray's Inn Road
London, WC1X 8DS
UK
Tel: 020 7794 5999
Fax: 020 7794 4702
Email: mail@lhc.org.uk
www.lhc.org.uk

(26) Tracy Longdon
21 Locksgreen Crescent,
Swindon
Wiltshire, SN25 3HR
UK
Tel: 01793 338791
Email: tracy@tracylongdonconsulting.co.uk
www.tracylongdonconsulting.co.uk

(27) Stella Martin (Heather Willings Health Through The Eyes
Cards)
19 The Broadway
Chichester
West Sussex, PO19 4QR
UK
Tel: 01243 781379

(28) Neutralec Ltd.
PO Box 2, Kidderminster
Worcestershire, DY11 6ZA
UK
Tel/Fax: 01562 823824
www.neutralec.com

(29) Powerwatch
2 Tower Road
Sutton, Ely
Cambridgeshire
CB6 2QA
UK
www.powerwatch.org.uk

(30) Roy & Ann Procter
Coombe Quarry
Keinton Mandeville
Near Somerton
Somerset, TA11 6DQ
UK
Fax: 01458 224234
Email: procter@dial.pipex.com
www.dspace.dial.pipex.com/procter

(31) Mike & Maureen Rawles
Westport
Somerset, TA10 0BN
UK
Tel: 01460-281450
www.dragonstone-uk.com

(32) Alfred Riggs
52 Sir John Fogge Avenue
Repton Park
Kent, TN23 3GA
United Kingdom
Tel: 01233 620036
Email: info@alfredriggs.com
www.alfredriggs.com

(33) Christopher & Veronika Strong
Stepping Stones
P.O. Box 108
Evesham, WR11 8ZL
UK
Tel: 01386 833899
Christopher.ssitu@btopenworld.com

(34) Subtle Field Technologies (Gary Johnson)
61 Tey Road., Earls Colne
Essex CO6 2LQ
UK
Tel: 01787 224377
Email: enquiries@subtlefieldtechnologies.com
www.subtlefieldtechnologies.com

(35) Svenska Slagruteforbundet (Swedish Society Of Dowsers)
Tel: 08 758 55 90
Email: ordforande@slagruta.org
www.slagruta.org

(36) Jane Thurnell-Read
Sea View House,
Long Rock, Penzance
Cornwall, TR 20 8JF
UK
Email: jane@lifeworkpotential.com
www.lifeworkpotential.com

(37) Transform Plus (Life Transformers)
2 The Cloisters, South Gosforth
Newcastle-upon-Tyne, NE7 7LS
UK
Tel: 0191 284 7615
christinefowler@yahoo.co.uk

(38) Pat Ward
5 Strathmore Close
Carterton
Oxfordshire, OX18 1FB
Email: tricia_ward@tiscali.co.uk

(39) Wholistic Research Company (Pulsor distributor)
Unit 1, Five House Farm
Sandon Road
Therfield, Royston
Hertfordshire, SG8 9RE
UK
Tel: 01763 284910
Fax: 01763 287467
Email: info@wholisticresearch.com
www.wholisticresearch.com
Also see www.pulsor.org

Printed in the United Kingdom
by Lightning Source UK Ltd.
124425UK00003B/187-189/A